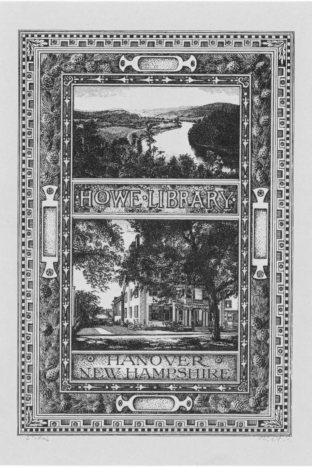

THE HEALING
COMPANION

THE HEALING
COMPANION

Simple and Effective Ways Your
Presence Can Help People Heal

JEFF KANE, M.D.

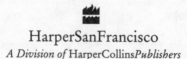

HarperSanFrancisco
A Division of HarperCollins*Publishers*

HarperCollins books may be purchased for educational, business, or sales promotional use. For information please write: Special Markets Department, HarperCollins Publishers, 10 East 53rd Street, New York, NY 10022.

HarperCollins Web site: http://www.harpercollins.com

HarperCollins®, ⚏®, and HarperSanFrancisco™ are trademarks of HarperCollins Publishers, Inc.

FIRST EDITION

Designed by Jessica Shatan

Library of Congress Cataloging-in-Publication Data
Kane, Jeff.
The healing companion : simple and effective ways your presence can help people heal / Jeff Kane.—1st ed.
p. cm.
Includes bibliographical references.
ISBN 0–06–251663–9 (cloth)
ISBN 0–06–251664–7 (paperback)
1. Death—Psychological aspects. 2. Care of the sick. 3. Terminally ill—Psychology. 4. Terminally ill—Family relationship. I. Title.
BF789.D4 K35 2001
649.dc21   00–033608

01 02 03 04 05 ❖ RRD(H) 10 9 8 7 6 5 4 3 2 1

To Gertrude Dorothy Kane
1905–1962

CONTENTS

FOREWORD

When I was in medical school, "healing" was considered something a wound did, not an event that was actually experienced by a human being. Healing, we medical students were told, was simply an automatic process lodged in the invisible recesses of the body's machinery, a process that had no connection with thought, feeling, or emotion. Similarly, the term *healer* did not arise in the course of our education. In fact, if someone had actually called us "healers," we would not have known whether we were being praised or damned. Looking back, I wish I'd had professors in medical school like Jeff Kane, M.D., who knows as much about genuine healing as any physician I've ever met.

How did we lose contact with healing? Whatever happened to healers? We sent them packing in the early days of the twentieth century and replaced them with a dazzling array of tools—vaccines, drugs, and surgical procedures. As medicine became increasingly high-tech, we thought we didn't need healing and healers any longer, and these concepts almost vanished from the vocabulary of medicine.

It is interesting to look back to see what we forgot. An example of a true healer is Sir William Osler (1849–1919), the

most influential physician in the history of modern medicine.[1]
After revolutionizing how medicine was taught and practiced in
the United States and Canada, in 1905, at the peak of his fame,
Osler was lured to England, where he became the Regius professor of medicine at Oxford. One day he went to graduation cere-
monies at Oxford, wearing his academic robes. On the way he
stopped by the home of his friend and colleague Ernest Mallam. One of Mallam's young sons was quite sick with whooping
cough and bronchitis. The child appeared to be dying, and he
would not respond to the ministrations of his parents or the
nurses. Osler loved children greatly, and he had a special way
with them. He would often play with them, and children would
invariably admit him into their world. So when Osler appeared
in his ceremonial robes, the little boy was captivated. After a
brief examination, Osler peeled a peach, cut and sugared it, and
fed it bit by bit to the enthralled patient. Although he felt recovery was unlikely, Osler returned for the next forty days, each
time dressed in his robes, and personally fed the young child
nourishment. Within just a few days the tide had turned and the
little boy's recovery became obvious—a recovery made possible
because Osler was a genius of a healer.

Today, new Oslers such as Jeff Kane are arising, and healing
is returning once again to medicine. As evidence, an increasing
number of medical schools are making a place for the importance of *meaning* in getting well. Consider the respect now being
given to the role of *spiritual* meaning. A decade ago almost no
medical schools taught students about the influence of spiritual
meaning in health. As of this writing, however, more than sixty
of the nation's 125 medical schools have formal courses exploring the role of spiritual meaning in health and illness.

The reasons that healing is returning to medicine are many.

For one thing, an increasing amount of scientific evidence shows that our thoughts, emotions, and perceived meanings can dramatically influence our physiology and make the difference in life and death. For another, the public is demanding a return of meaning to medicine, and this has given new status to healing.

Consider, for example, the movement toward complementary or alternative medicine (CAM). Currently, more Americans visit alternative practitioners annually than go to front-line, conventional physicians. By any measure, this is one of the most remarkable trends in our culture. Why is it happening? Dr. John Astin of Stanford University School of Medicine discovered in a recent national survey that people opt for complementary or alternative medicine largely because of spiritual reasons.[2] They believe that CAM-type therapies are more compatible with their inner beliefs than are conventional approaches. The trend toward complementary or alternative medicine, therefore, is a demand for a return of healers and genuine healing, which for most people is connected with spirituality and the honoring of one's inner life.

To understand healing, we have to shift gears in how we think about the practice of medicine. Modern medicine has become an exercise in *doing*, while healing is mainly a matter of *being*. Healing isn't something that can be practiced only by someone in a white coat; it can be practiced by anyone who is compassionately concerned about the welfare of another. While not just anyone can be a brain surgeon, everyone can be a healer. All that's required is love and caring, and paying attention to certain principles explained by Dr. Kane.

Without the peace and serenity that are the hallmark of true healing, conventional medical techniques will not work as well as they might. So, to those who may consider healing too soft a concept for our high-tech age, think again. Healing is not a luxury in medicine; it is a necessity. Healing is not the end of scientific medicine, but its fulfillment.

Everyone—patients and physicians alike—should be grateful to Dr. Jeff Kane for bringing the ancient wisdom of healing to light.

LARRY DOSSEY, M.D.
Author, *Reinventing Medicine* and *Healing Words*
Executive Editor, *Alternative Therapies in Health and Medicine*

In 1976, after practicing medicine for almost a decade, I realized that while I knew a fair amount about diseases, I had barely a clue as to how patients experienced sickness. Suspecting that healing was related less to diseases than to the people who manifested them, that gap bothered me.

Did I say *bothered?* No, it *obsessed* me to the point that I finally left my practice and instead invited patients to tell me what it was like to be sick. They received their medical care from other physicians and met with me in groups simply to speak. Such conversations have come to be known as "patient support groups."

Support group members usually begin by discussing their most obvious mutual concern, their disease. Those who have cancer speak about their tumors, X-rays, and blood tests. Those with AIDS speak of their infections, and those with lupus, their frayed physiologies. As they spend time together, grow closer, and listen more carefully, they discover a deeper commonality: recognition of their impermanence.

Of course, everyone's days are numbered, but a serious diagnosis certifies the fact. Participants quickly comprehend that whatever they are to do in this life, they'd better do it now. Their conversation inevitably shifts toward their passions and priorities, and soon tales of growth begin to replace those of suffering.

Virtually anyone is capable of initiating this process. We— the relatives, friends, and practitioners—who surround sick people can lift much of their load using nothing more than our full, honest presence. To do so is simple but not easy. In fact, it's a skill. This book will teach you how to be a *healing companion.*

An editorial note . . .

To protect the privacy of those whose stories I'll tell, I'll sometimes change their age and gender. And speaking of gender, I'll address the generic third person in a way you might find unusual. Common usage—"he"—rubs me the wrong way. On the other hand, when I use "she," female friends complain that women are portrayed as patients disproportionately. The neutral "they" and politically correct "he/she" feel artificial to me. So I've decided to use the masculine term in odd chapters and the feminine in even ones.

JEFF KANE, M.D.
Nevada City, California
June 2000

ACKNOWLEDGMENTS

The Healing Companion was generated by hundreds of support group members, principally at two northern California cancer centers, Sutter in Sacramento and Sierra Nevada in Grass Valley. They expressed their suffering, explored it, and ultimately teased wisdom and serenity from it. I watched, usually inspired and often astonished, and then went home and wrote it down. I offer them my ultimate compliment: they made me wonder.

Twenty years ago, medical colleagues to whom I mentioned support work looked at me as though I had a brain parasite. But times have changed, as they always do. Today I'm no longer lonely; indeed, physicians who treat the soul along with the body make up a major current in the professional mainstream. Healers, authors, and friends Marty Rossman, Rachel Naomi Remen, Larry Dossey, Bernie Siegel, Jerry Jampolsky, Andrew Weil, Bill Stewart, Maxine Barish, Jon Hake, Heath Foxlee, Brad Miller, Judi Wright, Scott Kellermann, and Dan Bibelheimer are rehumanizing healthcare as I write.

Sierra Nevada Cancer Center couldn't be more nurturing. Its medical director, Dr. Bill Newsom, and administrator, Ayse Turk-seven, have enthusiastically implemented my every suggestion. Its staff members, particularly Rebecca McCoy, Donna Fry, Jeanine Bryant, and Netta Kandell, are a joy to work with.

I offer thanks to my agent, Agnes Birnbaum, for her gentle humor and professional astuteness. Doug Abrams and his colleague at HarperSanFrancisco, Renee Sedliar, are fine editors, to be sure, but in addition, their warmth and flexibility lightened my writing task. They're also uncommonly focused people; if I digress or fulminate in this book, I do so despite their heroic efforts to keep me on track.

Thanks also to my writing group of the past six years— Valerie Kack-Brice, Sandra Rockman, Jeff Hattem, Jacquie Bellon, Liz Collins, and Ronnie Paul. I've benefited from their ideas, their encouragement, and their cast-iron patience with my interminable drafts.

I couldn't effectively engage seriously sick people without my own spiritual practice. I'm immensely grateful to yoga instructors Donald Moyer and Rama Vernon and their teacher, B. K. S. Iyengar; vipassana teacher Dr. Thynn Thynn, and my Tuesday meditation buddies; cartoon philosopher R. Crumb; and the many others who've led me, often kicking and screaming, toward mindfulness.

Most fundamentally, I thank my family. My parents provided me a safe and secure base. My wife, Ronnie Paul, hatha yoga teacher and Olympic-level existential cheerleader, maintains faith in me beyond all reason. And she and our daughters, Alix and Tashie, continually remind me of what's important.

THE HEALING
COMPANION

ONE

HEALING

> *There's a crucial difference between curing*
> *a disease and healing a person.*

We are healed of suffering only by experiencing it to the full.

—Marcel Proust

WHEN LOVED ONES SUFFER

I began to learn about healing the hard way when my aunt Gertie lay dying.

If I exhibit any cultural veneer whatever, I owe her the credit. Were it not for Gertie, I'd have little more in my head than medical data scattered around a field of baseball trivia. A former teacher, she made it her business to drag me weekly to Kabuki theater, Mr. Blackstone's magic show, Pete Seeger concerts. When I'd turn on the television, she'd reflexively turn it off and for good measure pull the plug.

"I think you'll read a book," she'd say.

After she became sick, Gertie, normally a feisty free spirit, played the good patient. She quietly acceded to a half-dozen operations, some of which I recognize today as predictably futile.

She acquiesced as well to the silence surrounding her sickness. Equated with doom in the public mind, cancer was in the early 1960s taboo par excellence. Even cannibalism was a more welcome topic of conversation. Those who suffered with cancer suffered alone. Gertie's pain was only partly in her body, then, and the rest was in her fear and isolation. However cancer savaged her flesh, it was loneliness and hopelessness that shattered her soul. She was only fifty-six years old when she died from The Disease with No Name.

Watching her shrink away, I ached for her and, to my surprise, for myself as well. I felt confused and angry even beyond my customary adolescent tumult. I couldn't fathom why no one would speak openly about what was obviously happening, and why my questions about it were answered with mumbles.

I was angry at our family's impotence. As much as we longed for something to say or do that might make Gertie feel a little better, we hadn't the slightest notion of direction, so when we were with her we sat with frozen faces, afraid to talk, let alone cry. In the end, for all the healing presence we mustered, we might as well have been cardboard silhouettes.

In hindsight, there was much we could have done. Today we call the relatives and friends of sick people *caregivers.* I like that term. It suggests that we who gather around the bedside aren't passive observers but can actually give care. Such skills are now available for the learning. If Gertie were sick today, at the very least we could avoid compounding her suffering with silence and fear. We'd ask her what was bothering her and discuss every emergent issue. We'd hold her hand, see to it that another heart was always cradling hers. Gradually, as we applied our skills, her fear and loneliness would drop away, and she could attain peace.

This book will guide you toward offering sick loved ones your healing presence. By learning to ask them exactly how they're suffering and help them express their feelings thoroughly, you'll encourage an atmosphere of honesty. You'll move toward a perspective in which *whatever* happens physically, the emotional turmoil surrounding it will settle. All involved will benefit from increasing serenity.

Helping sick people feel better can seem at first glance a trivial achievement compared to, say, eradicating their diseases or extending their lives. But presumably they've already hired experts toward those ends. Whether those practitioners succeed or not, your loved ones are suffering now, so I can't imagine anything of greater immediate value than helping alleviate that suffering. While your efforts may seem small, it is exactly these mundane acts—the hug, the glance, the open ear, the kind word—that serve as pivots around which lives rotate. Mother Teresa said, "You can't do great things; you can only do small things with love."

RELATIVES AND FRIENDS OF SICK PEOPLE SUFFER AND ARE TREATABLE

The small things that you can do for your sick loved ones will benefit you as well, since you're probably suffering, too. Obvious though it is that sickness is *emotionally* contagious, I never heard that in my medical training. I entered practice competent to diagnose and treat sick people, period. Their friends' and relatives' suffering was unfortunate, but outside my jurisdiction.

Now, though, I know otherwise. It feels entirely appropriate when the cancer patient's spouse, the parents of a sick child, the adult children of a dying elder pull me aside and whisper,

"What can I say? What can I do?" They ache to help, as I once ached. Feeling helpless, desperate, sad, angry, frustrated, and confused, they sense that what will alleviate their loved one's suffering might equally alleviate their own, and they're absolutely right.

A healing atmosphere is like fresh air: everyone breathes better. When my friend Christine learned she had breast cancer, the first person she told was her boyfriend, Al, with whom she'd lived for two years.

"Oh," Al said, "I guess we'll just do what we have to do about it," and turned to leave the room.

Christine was horrified. "Wait," she said. "I didn't just tell you the kitchen sink is clogged. I said I have cancer."

He wheeled around, snapping, "Well, what do you want me to do about it? You saw a doctor, didn't you?"

Christine was shocked speechless. She went upstairs, drew herself a hot bath, and cried in it for an hour. That evening she walked down the block to see her friend Anne. Alarmed at Christine's distress, Anne sat her down, made her a cup of tea, and asked her to describe everything that had happened.

"Christine," Anne said afterward, "I don't know Al to be like that. What do you think is going on with him?"

"I'm not sure. He's a kind man. That's what's so strange. He's even been around cancer before. He took care of his wife till she died of it." Seeing Anne's jaw drop, Christine paused thoughtfully. "Oh. I'll bet he's scared."

Christine didn't talk to Al about her cancer for the next week. She did, however, learn of a local support group for relatives of people with cancer. One morning she said to Al, "Honey, I haven't mentioned my cancer for a while. I know you're concerned about me, and I just want to let you know I'm doing okay."

"I'm glad to hear that."

"How are *you* doing?"

"Fine."

"Are you?" She looked him in the eye. "Tell me, do you think about Kate these days?"

Al's eyes filled with tears. Then he broke into a shaking sob. Christine put her arms around him. Her face beside his, she whispered, "You know, I think you're hurting more than I am. There's nothing wrong with you for hurting, or for letting me know it. In fact, it makes me love you all the more."

They spoke for an hour. Al admitted that when Christine had given him the news of her cancer, he'd felt absolutely crushed, but he thought saying so would injure her spirits. She said, "Well, maybe you're right. Maybe you should talk to someone else about it." She told him about the relatives' group.

Al says, "So I went to the group. I imagined it'd be a bunch of whiners sobbing to each other. But it was just normal people, all kinds. They asked me what I'd like to say. I said there wasn't much to say. A man sitting across from me, nice guy about my age, said, 'Al, that was the first thing I said here, too, not much to say. Takes guys like us a little while to clear our throats, right? I held it in awhile, then, boy, I spoke. Can't stop me now.'

"Well, he was right. Next time I went, I said that when Christine told me she had cancer, that moment had to be the bottom of my life, even worse than when my wife was sick. The guy asked me, 'Sick with what?' and I said, 'Breast cancer, like Christine has now.'

"Well, there were gasps and rolling eyes. Just about everybody in the room said, 'No wonder,' and then it all came together for me. I thought I'd finished with pain over Kate's death, but apparently not."

As Al attended group sessions over the next month, he learned a great deal about himself, especially his anger, fear, and grief.

"I was so scared when Kate was sick," he says. "I thought if I told her how I felt, it'd bring her down. I thought if I spoke to her about the possibility she'd die—which was always on my mind—it would somehow make it happen. Maybe she felt the same way. I really don't know because we didn't speak. Both of us were so frightened of so many things, we were paralyzed. Now I realize life doesn't have to be that way. I know more now; maybe I'm wiser. My group's helped me understand my experience with Kate.

"Just a few nights ago, I asked Christine how she was doing, and she said she was thinking about death. Well, that's always been a morbid subject in my book. But my support group encourages me to question every bit of fear I find, so I won't go through this with Christine like I did with Kate. I sat with her remark for a minute, going through all sorts of mental acrobatics, and finally said to her, 'What about death?'

"She said, 'You know, Al, everybody dies sometime.'

"'I know,' I said.

"'That means we're all going to lose one another. We came here alone and we'll leave alone. There's no way around it.'

"I'd never thought about it quite like that. 'Yeah, you're right,' I said, and sat with it some more. 'I'm not sure what that means to me,' I finally said. 'What do you make of it?'

"Christine hugged me close and said, 'It means we'd better love one another the best we can right now.'

"Whew! She's so right. I'm closer with Christine at this point than I've ever been with anyone, but I'll go for more, too. It's not enough for her and me to just say our stuff. We take it further, ask each other what we mean, clarify until we really understand what we're talking about. Maybe these are the first real conversations I've ever had. If there's anything we haven't talked about, I'd like to know what it is. She's got cancer, sure, but she's also got me and I've got her."

How Sick People Suffer

A quarter-century ago, I steered my medical practice in an unusual direction. Instead of only diagnosing and treating people, I began to listen fully to them. Although I'd been trained to harvest diagnostic clues from a patient's narrative and ignore the rest, now I strained to hear it all.

When I listened in this way, I heard their fears, anxieties, confusion, depression, and rages. In other words, I heard their suffering in detail. I learned that people get emotional when they're sick, and that fear and anger and despair aren't abnormal; they're a natural feature of sickness. In fact, I'd worry about the mental health of sick people who *weren't* affected by their consequent feelings.

Hearing many hundreds of stories, I gradually learned that people don't generally suffer from their disease as much as from their emotions, the reactions their disease ignites in them. (Most of those with whom I work have cancer, but what I'll say in this book applies as well to people with other diagnoses.) This revelation surprised me as much as it probably does you. But think about it. Recall what bothered you when you were last sick. I'll wager that your physical disease, the abnormality in structure or function, didn't disturb you anything like the disease's effects on your *experience*—your pain and fear, your anger, inconvenience, frustration, grief, or some other essentially emotional process.

You might be tempted to assume I'm saying your suffering was "all in your head." No. On the contrary, it was all too real. Experience, including suffering, which I'll discuss in the next chapter, is every bit as real, and at least as treatable, as physical disease.

When I first explored how people experienced serious sickness, I naively asked them, "What bothers you about your cancer?" Those who took my question seriously and followed it to its logical extent offered answers that were arrestingly unique to each.

"It means I'm going to die."

"I have to accept other people's help."

"I can't stand pity."

"My privacy will be violated."

"I don't mind dying, but I don't think I can handle . . ."

". . . the pain."

". . . the expense."

". . . the treatment."

". . . disfigurement."

". . . becoming a vegetable."

". . . leaving my family."

". . . loss of control."

We naturally make assumptions about what sick people must be experiencing, but we actually have no idea what's going on inside them *unless we ask*, since sickness is intensely personal. Two people with identical diagnoses share only the physical disorder; the way they experience that disorder is absolutely unique to each. They'll find different meanings in their sickness, feel different emotions, respond with different behaviors.

They not only suffer individually but in ways that vary by the day and hour as well. If you ask, "What bothers you about your cancer *right now*?" you can expect a curiously ordinary answer.

Sick people aren't plagued from moment to moment by vast existential issues as much as by the trials of daily life.

One person complains, "I'm angry at my doctor. He never gives me any time."

Another says, "My recent surgery's left me too tired to drive. My wife has to ferry the kids, so I feel useless."

"Chemotherapy numbed my tongue, so my favorite foods taste like cardboard."

Once people express their suffering with this specificity, they usually find their own methods for dealing with it. My friend Gene, who had widespread kidney cancer, was chatting one evening with his wife, Rose.

"So," she said, "how are you doing?"

He mused, "You know, something astonishes me. It seems like I ought to feel worse about my cancer. You know, depressed or fearful, maybe. But I really don't. There's no pain. I don't feel scared of dying. Isn't that strange?"

"Well, does *anything* bother you?"

He thought about it. "Hmmm. As a matter of fact, my weight loss does. Look at me." He stood and extended his arms. "Isn't this just pathetic? I'm as skinny as a rail. Now that is driving me up the wall. I can't stand to look like a scarecrow."

"Did you tell the doctor?"

"Sure, but he said weight loss comes with cancer."

"This woman in my office, Jenny, sure wishes she had your problem," Rose said. "She's gaining weight like mad. Says it's a side effect of some medicine for her breast cancer."

"Hmmm," Gene said, "can you ask her what it is?"

When he next saw his doctor, Gene requested that medicine. The doctor objected, "That's a female hormone. It's not for you."

"You don't understand. This weight loss is damaging my will to live."

That was all the doctor needed to hear. He wrote the prescription, and three weeks later, Gene grinned as he told Rose, "Just weighed myself. Eighteen pounds up!"

Gene's distress over his weight loss was gone. It was that simple. Rose did nothing more complicated than ask him exactly how his cancer disturbed him, and Gene took it from there.

Suffering intolerable weight loss or dependency on others or losing one's sense of taste may sound like minor complaints compared to the overall stakes, but day by day, they're what serious sickness is usually about.

WHAT HEALING IS

If you're to heal with your presence, you need to know exactly what healing is—and is not. Healing is best described as *the attainment of inner peace.* As such, it's not the same as curing, which is a physical process, the restoration of normal tissue. We confuse healing with curing as routinely as we blur love with sex, and with equally troublesome results. By comparing the two concepts, we can understand each better.

Curing and healing are both essential to our well-being, since every sick person lives with both his physical disease and his simultaneous emotional experience of the disease. I'm not saying anything new here. Since the 1970s, a growing number of medical authors—including Joan Borysenko, Deepak Chopra, Larry Dossey, Jerry Jampolsky, Elisabeth Kübler-Ross, Lawrence LeShan, Rachel Naomi Remen, Martin Rossman, Oliver Sacks, Bernie Siegel, Abraham Verghese, and Andrew Weil—have reaffirmed the notion that sickness affects both body and mind.

Obvious though this sounds, it means something quite strik-
ing: sickness isn't a single process but two simultaneous ones.
Sickness alters the way our bodies function, and it also makes us
feel terrible. These authors call the physical aspect of sickness
disease and the personal experience of the sickness *illness.* They
generally agree that while we're fairly adept at treating physical
disease, we're relatively backward at treating illness.

To address the latter effectively, we'll need to further clarify
the distinction. The "disease" is a tangible, measurable event,
amenable to medical science's manipulations. The sick person's
experience of being sick, his "illness," isn't a physical, visible, measurable phenomenon, but it's no less real than disease.

With cancer, for example, the disease consists of the
tumor—its location, size, stage, cellular characteristics, X-ray
findings, and so on. In the case of diabetes, the disease includes
serum sugar–level abnormalities and blood vessel blockage. In
heart disease, it can be an erratic pulse or deformed valve.

In contrast, the experience of being sick is just that, experience. "Illness" includes, then, the sick person's fear, anxiety, depression, anger, isolation, despair, and so on—in other words,
his suffering.

We doctors are well trained to treat physical disease. We can
set broken limbs, prescribe appropriate antibiotics, and remove
diseased organs. These endeavors can possibly lead to a cure, de-
fined as eradication of the disease.

But we can't cure fear or some other species of suffering, because suffering exists outside the realm of the physically man-
ageable. Of course, we can prescribe a pill that offers temporary
relief from suffering, but we can't make it go away.

Diseases, then, may be cured, but only people are healed. They're healed
when they experience their suffering and make their way

through it as skillfully as possible, and it is toward this process that you'll direct your efforts.

In her landmark book *On Death and Dying,* Dr. Elisabeth Kübler-Ross listed a number of emotions that people experience when they confront their mortality. They deny, get angry, bargain frantically, get depressed. When they finish expressing whatever arose, when their emotional froth has boiled off and none is left, they simply feel quiet. You may have noticed this kind of peace yourself after your last "good cry," when you felt drained and tired, but finished, complete.

Kübler-Ross called this state, the last item on her list, *acceptance.* Acceptance isn't an emotion at all; on the contrary, it is the absence of emotion.

HEALING AS EQUANIMITY

Your sick friend or relative is healed when he reaches the point of acceptance, which is the same as equanimity. The healed state by definition concerns only his present moment. Thus equanimity isn't the same as resignation, his anticipation of a pessimistic future. Nor does it involve considerations of the past, including, say, a quest for the cause of his disease. The healed state is neither more nor less than calm acceptance of his immediate situation.

You can guide him to this destination by being skillfully present, which means offering him a special kind of attention.

Healing attention emphasizes listening over speaking, a tilt that may surprise you. We generally assume that what makes a difference lies in what we say rather than in what we hear. The most frequent question I'm asked by friends and relatives of sick people is "What can I say?" There's agony behind this, since they correctly suspect hollowness in exhortations like "Hang in there," "I just know you're going to beat this," and "If you've got to have cancer, then this is the kind to get."

They're usually relieved to hear that they needn't say any-thing, only listen. After all, they can't begin to alleviate the sick person's suffering until they know what it consists of, how he hurts right now, and they can't know that unless they ask. In fact, the sick person often isn't fully aware of it himself until he articulates it.

My friend Rita and her daughter Penny illustrate this process nicely. Rita had lung cancer eight years ago. Following surgery, she went into remission for five years, a delightful surprise for Rita and her doctor as well. She moved hundreds of miles to be with Penny, but then, over the next several months, felt increas-ingly tired and short of breath. Having secured no local doctor yet, she had Penny drive her to an emergency room. There it was discovered that her cancer had returned. This time it was a mass that filled her pericardium, the sac around her heart.

"I didn't know then that my life was threatened," Rita says, "but I learned it right away when I watched the doctors. Faces don't lie, and each doctor looked graver than the last. I knew I was in big trouble."

Dr. Morton, a heart surgeon, confirmed to Rita that she was indeed teetering on the edge. He operated that day, removing the tumor and her pericardium along with it.

Rita awoke in the intensive care unit with Penny at her bed-side. Her anesthesia cleared over the next twelve hours, and she was finally able to speak.

The first thing she said was "I'm afraid."

"But I think you're out of the woods now, Mom."

"I'm really afraid, anyway."

Penny considered this. "Can you say more?"

Rita began to speak about her discomfort. Initially she rambled, as she was in pain and still somewhat disoriented by drugs she'd been given, but at last was able to say, "I think people here won't know who I am."

"What do you mean?"

Rita looked Penny in the eye. "Honey, I'm special. I'm strong, a fighter. I've survived diseases and treatments people die from all the time. I'm new here, and people don't know me. They might think I'm just an average patient and give up on me."

She soon fell asleep. Penny phoned Dr. Morton and told him what Rita had said.

Late that evening he came to her bedside, sat, took her hand, and said, "I received your medical records and read them. By God, you accomplished the unexpected before, and I think maybe you can do it again."

"How I needed to hear that!" Rita says now. "That nubbin of hope was my turning point. My fear just melted away." Three years later, she remains free of cancer and leads a satisfying life.

Rita underwent a simultaneous pair of experiences, her physical disease—her tumor—and her illness—her panic that she wouldn't be recognized for who she was. Fortunately, Penny helped her clarify the latter, and Dr. Morton addressed it successfully. Rita was *cured*, at least for the present, of her tumor; and by being recognized, she was *healed*.

DYING DOESN'T PRECLUDE HEALING

Uncomfortable with the concept of death, our culture pushes us to conceive of survival as "winning" and dying as "losing." We easily assume, then, that healing and dying are mutually exclusive. If this pattern lurks within your own thinking, I suggest dropping it, since a dying person can indeed heal.

Healing is an internal experience, so it's untethered to physical time and space. It's similar in that way to imagination, the domain of all possibilities, which of course includes the impossible. Unlinked as it is to any physical condition, then, there's no reason that healing can't occur even as one gets sicker and dies.

But let's back up a step: how do we even know when someone is "dying" or, for that matter, "terminal"? Having been in this business awhile, I'm still fooled more often than not: healthy friends suddenly perish, and the critically sick miraculously rebound. All we can be sure of is that every sick person is alive and will eventually die. We can certify that someone was dying only after he has died. Even when we suspect his end is near, he is still living, and so subject to suffering and hopefully to its alleviation.

Liz and Clarence were in their late seventies, and both had cancer. Married for more than fifty years and with no children, they were supremely devoted to each other. Liz's cancer began to gallop such that she needed to be hospitalized. Every day Clarence sat by her bed from dawn until late at night. The nurses on all shifts came to love them both.

After two weeks, Liz began drifting in and out of a coma. Clarence continued to attend her, brightening when she was lucid and becoming despondent when she floated away. The head nurse, Stevie, told one of her subordinates, "I've seen a whole lot of people die, and it's plain to me that Liz won't go while Clarence is with her. She needs a little time to herself."

Early one morning, Stevie advised Clarence, "You know, it's not helping you or Liz to exhaust yourself like this, Clarence. Why don't you go down to the cafeteria and get some breakfast? We'll keep a close eye on Liz, I promise."

While Clarence was at breakfast, Stevie sat with Liz, stroking her hand. Liz awoke. "I'm still here," she smiled at Stevie. "Where's Clarence?"

"Clarence left to have breakfast. There's only me here with you now, and I'll stay."

Squeezing Stevie's fingers, Liz said, "How I love him." She closed her eyes, and in a few minutes her heart stopped.

The standard nursing procedure at this point was to close the curtains around Liz's bed and prepare her body, which included removing her jewelry for safekeeping. But Stevie couldn't dislodge Liz's wedding ring. She tried wetting the finger, and then massaged it with a lubricant, all to no avail. The ring stayed obstinately put, and Stevie gave up.

When Clarence returned, Stevie met him, put her hands on his shoulders, and told him that Liz had died.

Clarence nodded, bent his head. "I'd like a few minutes with her." He entered the curtained-off area.

Stevie went about her business and returned as Clarence was emerging from Liz's room. His hand was closed around something. Noting Stevie's curiosity, he opened his hand and there, on his palm, was Liz's wedding ring.

WHY WE NEED HEALING

As you learn healing skills, your sick loved one may reap an unexpected benefit. In addition to the relief of his suffering and yours, he may find that he no longer needs as much medical care.

Stanford University researchers discovered recently that arthritis support group participants utilized 40 percent less doctor time, even months after leaving their group. This and similar studies with similar conclusions help confirm my colleagues' perennial claim that a significant proportion of their patients don't have a medical problem as much as a social one that affects their bodies, and they need someone simply to listen to them and help them sort things out. Indeed, when Sigmund Freud was still a child, Viennese physician Rudolf Virchow, considered the father of modern pathology, remarked, "Much illness is a conflict in values sailing under a physiological flag."

If healing actually reduces the need for medical intervention—along with its hazards and expense—might it do even more? Might it also promote cure? That is, can alleviation of a patient's suffering act as partial treatment for his physical disease?

Cures certainly promote healing. Say I break my arm and am miserable from loss of its use. I feel angry about it, perhaps guilty, dependent, ashamed: that's my "illness." As the bone knits, the pain and disability gradually vanish. A year later, the fracture is cured and I'm no longer troubled in any way by it. When the injury-associated emotions depart, I'm healed.

Fascinatingly, the opposite is also true. Healing can indeed promote cure. We've known since the 1930s, from the research of Hans Selyé and others, that stress hobbles the immune system. We know that all else being equal, patients who feel hopeless and helpless will plummet, and those who feel hopeful and in control will do measurably better. So many studies support this conclusion that it's no longer controversial.

But how does it work? How can we explain scientifically how something as intangible as a patient's attitude can affect the course of his disease? Dr. Candace Pert, a former senior researcher at the National Institute of Mental Health, and others published a paper in the *Journal of Immunology*[1] about endorphins, potent painkilling hormones that naturally occur deep in the brain. Researchers already knew that receptors for endorphins— that is, the sites where these hormones have their effect—were located in the brain, but Pert and her colleagues found receptors *outside* the brain, too. Some were on the surface of white blood cells, which are responsible in part for disease resistance and tissue restoration.

In other words, a brain chemical associated with mood directly influences the immune system: Pert and her colleagues had found a molecular link between attitude and physiology, mind and body. Musing on the implications, Pert said: "The truth is so weird that I've only recently come to believe in it and experience it. . . . There's a wisdom in every cell. . . . Consciousness precedes matter. It's not like a peptide [brain chemical] creates the feeling. The feeling creates the peptide."[2]

The feeling creates the peptide: a revolutionary concept in medical science. Where we traditionally assume human behavior to result from arcane biochemistry, the opposite may be the case. As I subjectively feel better, my physiology acts more healthily. My immune system mimics my attitude. My protective cells and antibodies feel their oats when I do, and go slack when I feel helpless. In sum, as I heal, my body drives toward a cure. But you might have intuited this same conclusion with no research at all. Recalling your own experience, where would you predict your arthritis would be more likely to flare, at your child's wedding or your IRS audit?

Dr. Pert's research can help explain startling clinical revelations. Psychiatrist Dr. David Spiegel and his colleagues at Stanford University demonstrated a decade ago that women with breast cancer who participated in support groups (which treat members' feelings and attitudes, not their tumors) *doubled* their survival time over matched women who received only standard medical care.

Since then, however, other researchers have been unable to consistently replicate Spiegel's results. It may be that support group participants alter only their life quality, not necessarily its quantity. In any case, breast cancer expert Dr. Craig Henderson of the University of California, San Francisco, assesses the field this way: "If you proceed on the basis of the published literature, there is better evidence right now that psychosocial support extends survival time with breast cancer than there is similar evidence for bone marrow transplantation."[3]

HEALING IS EASY, BUT IT'S NOT SIMPLE

Although healing others is fairly easy, acquisition of the skill can be a thorny journey. We may encounter a substantial mental obstruction: the notion that the physical disease is the entire ball game. We might perceive the sick person's experience, his illness, as daunting, but still only an unfortunate side effect of the disease rather than an event of equal significance. Failing to value his illness fully, we'll see his treatment exclusively as the application of medical technology to the disease. Little wonder we can feel unqualified to work with sick people.

We're even bereft of the mental images that would allow us to consider healing coequal with curing. When I ask people to conjure images of healing, they usually produce pictures of stethoscopes, digital readouts, test tubes, scanners, and the like. These are uniformly pictures of medical technology, of tools for curing, not for healing.

If these are your images, console yourself with the knowledge that your limit isn't personal but cultural. A television station did a story on a cancer patient support group I facilitated. Nothing more intricate than conversation occurs in support groups. Our highest-tech equipment is Kleenex. When the story aired, the reporter introduced it with, "And now, some interesting medical news . . ." Behind her appeared a logo establishing the story's category. Was the logo a graphic of two people talking? Certainly not. It was a chest X-ray. After all, how would viewers know this was a medical story if not for the technological clue?

During the past two generations, our media have reinforced the notion that healthcare equals technology by enchanting us continually with high-tech breakthroughs—organ transplants, cloning, telemedicine, microsurgery. Some of this news amounts to hyperbole or outright marketing, to be sure, but having labored among the white-coated, I can tell you there's much to it. It works.

Relentless publicity of its glitter, though, has insidiously whittled our wider concept of healthcare as surely as water wears down stone. Whereas in the 1930s the word *doctor* evoked Norman Rockwell images of bedside concern, today the picture is of a clear-eyed scientist pushing buttons on a complex control panel, operating by robot on a patient a thousand miles away. Dr. Kildare has morphed into Captain Kirk.

To heal, then, begin to switch the flavor of your intent from high-tech to low-tech. In fact, I doubt that you can engage in anything less technical than healing, since its only tool is the relationship between you and your sick friend or relative. Anything you can possibly place between you in order to enhance contact—a machine, a chart, a crystal, software—can only haze the relationship and inadvertently impede healing.

You Can Make a Difference

Interestingly, your healing efforts will often accomplish even more than standard medical intervention will. You may not have known that the number of patient visits for incurable diseases now exceeds those for curable ones. Because of our sparkling successes in treating infectious diseases and trauma, people generally live longer—long enough, anyway, to develop the chronic

diseases of older age. The word *chronic*, meaning of long duration, happens to be a euphemism for *incurable*. All we can do
medically for the people who suffer chronic diseases—including
most arteriosclerosis, diabetes, arthritis, an array of autoim-
mune and neurologic diseases, and many cases of cancer—is to
try to slow the disease's progress and relieve symptoms. Our
most pressing healthcare challenge today can't be to cure these
diseases but to help people bear them with less suffering. Simply
put, we need a technology for healing, and we need it now.

Take heart as you embark on the healing quest, for the bulk
of our healthcare legacy, from Galen to Maimonides to
Nightingale to Schweitzer, is behind you. Until early in this century, healthcare was far less about technology than about the
healing relationship. Sir William Osler, the patriarch of North
American medicine, advised that it is "more important to know
what sort of patient has the disease than what sort of disease
the patient has." Modern medical science is a monument to
human will, wit, and craft, but it can't be the sole approach to
sick people. Sickness must be addressed technically *and* with an
intent to alleviate suffering. No one's forcing us to choose one
over the other. They're obligatory complements. Your sick friend
or relative needs his disease treated effectively, and he needs, in
equal measure, your healing presence.

TO HEAL

*1. Recognize that healing is the sick person's attainment of
equanimity,* whereas curing is resolution of his physical
disease. ✍

(continued)

2. Remembering that healing is your mission, attend to the person rather than to his disease. Learn what *disturbs* him about his disease. Ask "How does your sickness make you feel?" "What is it that bothers you about being sick?" and "How has your sickness affected your life?" ✐

3. Be hopeful: suffering is *always* treatable. ✐

TWO

ILLNESS

| A serious disease shatters the lives of both patients and those around them, and everyone *is healable*. |

Man is not disturbed by events, but by the view he takes of them.
—Epictetus (ca. A.D. 55–ca. 135)

NEWS OF SICKNESS IS DEVASTATING

In order to heal people, you'll need to see their illness—that is, their experience of sickness—as equal in significance to their physical disease. Even the onset of their illness, the moment they learn of their diagnosis, can be catastrophic.

Ellen found a lump in her breast. Frantic, she phoned Dr. Fry. When he saw her the following day he took a small specimen through a fine needle. Appreciating Ellen's anxiety, he promised he'd give her the biopsy results as soon as possible.

Ellen didn't sleep that night. Instead, she lay awake imagining the entire miserable gauntlet she was surely about to run. Veteran cancer patients, primed by their history to suspect the worst in any symptom, call this understandable exercise *awfulizing.*

The next afternoon, Ellen's phone rang. "Ellen, hi, this is Fran, Dr. Fry's nurse. We just received your biopsy results, and the doctor asked me to phone you with them. Your biopsy was negative."

"Oh. Well, thank you," Ellen answered, and hung up. She was stunned, having taken the message as confirmation of her most morbid fears. She had no idea "negative" meant *no* cancer was found.

In a few hours her husband, Dave, came home and found her staring silently. As he spoke with her, he realized Ellen wasn't sure where she was or even who she was. He rushed her to the local emergency room.

The physician on duty, learning that Ellen had recently had a breast biopsy, thought that her disorientation might represent a tumor that had spread to her brain. Among other tests, he performed a spinal tap to examine her spinal fluid. The tap proved normal, but Ellen suffered one of its common side effects, a monster headache. The doctor prescribed a pain medication to which Ellen was apparently hypersensitive, for she lost consciousness.

She awoke the next morning in the intensive care unit. A neurologist examined her there and afterward offered a startling diagnosis: transient global amnesia. "All that means," the doctor explained, "is that you were probably stressed something fierce, and it pretty literally blew your mind. In other words, no brain tumor, no disease. You can expect your memory to return within a few days."

Ellen now reflects, "I still can't believe all that happened to me. I wasn't sick with *anything,* but I felt like I'd been yanked out of my life and locked in a trunk. I'd hate to think what people go through who get diagnosed for real!"

Ellen's point is well taken. When people learn they're sick, the implications that occur to them—everything from annoyance to death—constitute a major life event. If it's never happened to you, then imagine the moment you learn you're seriously sick. I'll offer cancer as an example, but feel free to substitute another condition.

In a word, you're devastated.

Let's say the tumor was found early. At this point it's a little lump and has actually done no harm, but it naturally agitates you, since it's an omen of what might come. That is, *you're devastated not by the tumor but by the news.* This is the beginning of your illness, your personal experience of the disease you now know you have.

Devastation is more than an inconvenient appendage to the disease. The late Anatole Broyard, literary critic for the *New York Times,* wrote in *Intoxicated by My Illness* that discovery of his diagnosis disoriented him as though he'd been abducted across the border to a land whose terrain, customs, and language were a total mystery.

Try operating normally after you've been clicked a half-channel off as Broyard and my friend Ellen were. Your routines, your daily comforts, your plans are suddenly blown away like so much confetti. This is a profound loss, since one way of defining your very personality is as the aggregate of your habits. No wonder, then, that you sit confounded, wondering where the "you" that you've always known has gone. Since news of your sickness challenges your customary sense of self, now you're confronted with two issues: your serious physical disease and the revelation that you might be losing your mind.

Wander around your home and you'll find a further aggravation. Spreading to everyone within a hug's reach, news of your disease broadsides your family habits, mangles every dynamic. Within hours, no one's sure what's required. Can I speak about it? Can I cry openly? What can I do to help? What shouldn't I say? Dormant issues revive. Why wasn't it me? Isn't that just like her, to pick this week? Maybe now he'll think about someone besides himself. Suddenly the family acts like it's on the strings of a demented puppeteer.

The family's relationships are damaged, and so are the individuals themselves. If you're a caregiver, you may know firsthand that relatives and friends can suffer more visibly than the sick person does. Begin your healing work, then, by suspecting that the newly diagnosed person is devastated and possibly feeling deranged, and suspect as well that those around her may be similarly injured. Suffering is suffering, no matter who's called the patient.

Fortunately for my friend Jenny, her neighbor Charlotte saw clearly how the sick person isn't the only sufferer. After Jenny's husband, Ron, returned home from hospitalization for an AIDS-related infection, Jenny put him to bed and cared for him magnificently.

The first time Charlotte visited, she said, "Jenny, that sign at the front door, POSITIVE VIBES ONLY, what does that mean?"

"Oh, the books all say negativity damages people's immune systems. Why?"

"Well, I imagined visitors seeing that sign and putting on steel smiles, that's all."

"Well, yeah, sometimes you need to force positivity."

"Do *you?*"

Jenny's eyes watered. She moved her mouth but couldn't speak.

"Jenny, can we sit down?"

Jenny nodded, and she and Charlotte spent the rest of the afternoon talking. As she spoke, Jenny realized that whereas Ron was in decent spirits, her refusal to admit her own fear and anxiety had rendered her brittle.

She now says, "I couldn't have faked positivity much longer. I'd have cracked up, and then what sort of help would I have been for Ron? Charlotte and I spoke together several times after that, and each time I felt a little more settled and solid. I'm still in pain about Ron's AIDS, but I also take things a day at a time, feel more relaxed about it."

I learned in my medical training that cancer is a tumor, a heart attack is oxygen-starved cardiac muscle, AIDS is a perilous viral infection, Alzheimer's disease is gray-matter deterioration. True enough, but incomplete, like saying that Dracula is a Transylvanian. The picture of a serious sickness' full effect is more like a bomb detonating in the living room, leaving the home in debris and its occupants shredded.

The damage's duration depends largely on how well it's addressed. The period of initial wreckage lasts on the order of days to weeks, but longer in direct proportion to how thoroughly it's repressed or ignored. It's fair to inform newly sick families, though, that their turbulence (standardly called *the emotional roller coaster*) is definitely transient.

ATTENDING TO SUFFERING RATHER THAN DISEASE

When you observe sick loved ones, you might naturally assume that their physical disease is the source of their suffering. After all, if it weren't for the disease they'd probably feel fine. Yet they have it, and whether anyone can affect its course is unknowable. But you can do something about their suffering, so focus on that rather than on their physical situation.

My friend Morris saw his doctor for what he thought were minor symptoms. He emerged from the encounter with the stunning diagnosis of scleroderma: his immune system was attacking his own tissues.

As he went through further diagnostic procedures over the next two weeks, he was continually angry. "Why me?" he raged. "Why not my business partner, may his guts turn to stone?"

He vented his spleen on family, friends, doctors, and most understood. But when Morris remained no less volcanic two months into his treatment, his girlfriend, Susan, insisted that they discuss it.

"Morris, what's going on with you?"

"What's going on with me? Isn't it obvious? I have scleroderma!"

"I see two problems, Morris. One is your scleroderma, for sure. The other is this constant anger. And only the scleroderma's getting treated at this point." She paused. "Look, which one bothers you more right now?"

"If you think you're going to talk me out of being angry, you're nuts! I've got a right to be angry!"

Days later, Susan asked, "Morris, aren't you getting tired of being angry all the time?"

Suddenly sensing the energy he'd channeled into stoking his furnace, Morris burst into tears.

"I cried on and off most of that afternoon," he says. "Susan stayed with me, helped me get it all out. Afterward, I felt calmer than I have in years. I've still got scleroderma, and that's enough without ripping out my insides every day, too."

In discovering that his suffering was based not in his disease but in his illness, his anger in his case, Morris was able to express it honestly and fully, and so then attain some peace. His scleroderma wasn't cured, but Morris himself was healed.

WE GENERALLY SEE SUFFERING AS LESS SIGNIFICANT THAN DISEASE

Even when we witness firsthand the emotional carnage wrought by a serious sickness, we tend tenaciously to return our gaze to the physical disease. In Morris's case, for example, we might lament, Oh, poor Morris! His scleroderma makes him angry, and he inflicts that on everyone else. If we can put a man on the moon, why can't we find a cure for scleroderma?

Focusing on the disease will lead us to frustration sooner than to healing, but we choose it understandably: as a tangible, objectively verifiable event, Morris's disease seems more real than his illness. We can see it, point it out to one another, even measure it.

In contrast, we can't sense Morris's anger ourselves, only hear about it from him. It's not easy to communicate the subtle flavors and increments of suffering. Everyone who's ever hurt knows that some pains are worse than others, but when I ask a roomful of people, "Who here has had the worst pain?" they grin back at me. One usually jokes, "The worst pain is *my* pain." They're aware that the functions that make us human—pain, humor, fear, love—can never be objectively gauged.

In our science-venerating society, concrete events are afforded more credence than unverifiable experiences are. We can remove a kidney or a femur and exhibit it on a tray, but how can we display a measure of mind? Our inner life, admittedly not of the material world, can fairly be called immaterial, a word that also means irrelevant. If experience is ethereal, it seems unstable as well: thoughts and feelings rise and fall with less constancy than flames. In addition, experience seems so specific to each person, so unique, that I marvel whenever two people happen to understand each other.

Little wonder, then, that we favor the physical world as our prime indicator of reality. When faced with a conflict between objective data and our inner experience, we regularly favor the former.

My friend Pam had chronic hepatitis. She waved the results of her latest lab tests at her sister Chloe, who's a nurse. "Look at these, would you, please?" she said. "They don't make sense to me."

Chloe looked. A number of tests suggested that Pam's liver function was more impaired than ever. "How don't they make sense to you?"

"They're terrible. They say my liver's puny. But the fact is I feel fine."

"Pam, what bothers you about this?"

"How can I feel fine when these tests say otherwise? I can't feel good. I'm kidding myself. I'm in denial." She sank heavily into a chair.

Chloe sat beside her. They didn't speak for a minute. Then Pam said, "On the other hand, I feel like I feel. Matter of fact, all I've ever been sure of is how I feel. Why would I let numbers tell me I'm not feeling good when I do feel good? Why would I want to make myself feel bad? That's crazy."

I agree with her. Pam's liver is sick, but that doesn't negate the fact that she feels well. What would anyone accomplish by convincing her that her liver tests are more valid than her feelings? My inner cynic might inform me that she won't feel well for long, but that's all the more reason she should honor her current feelings.

Fortunately, only in public do we allow abstractions like numbers to refute what we actually feel. Though we openly advise one another, "Now, don't let your emotions decide this.

Try to be objective," in our heart of hearts, feelings nevertheless hold sway. We make our most important decisions—whom to marry or divorce, which job to take or quit, when to embark on an adventure—emotionally, a strategy that serves as well as any. However we outwardly extol rationality as the sail of our ship, below the waterline our dreamworld remains the rudder. We can endorse objectivity all we like, but as Epictetus observed, we'll inevitably respond to what we make of events rather than to the events themselves. We act from meaning more than from fact. In the sense that our inner world actually dominates our outer, we'd do well to stop considering imagination imaginary.

Even we doctors, allegedly hard-nosed scientists, routinely listen to our guts. I've made it a point for years to ask my colleagues—outside the hearing range of attorneys, of course—if they've ever made a medical decision from a "hunch" that contradicted their data. One hundred percent whisper in the affirmative.

ILLNESS IS AS REAL AS DISEASE

Despite popular credence in fact over feeling, our inner world may actually be *more* reliable than our outer. Our case in point, physical disease, has shifted its shape constantly through history, whereas experience of it has persisted relatively unchanged.

Mutating germs, cumulative environmental toxins, and extended lifespans inevitably sprout new diseases—consider AIDS and Legionnaire's disease—while some others, such as smallpox and scurvy, become rare or extinct. Sometimes we decide that diseases are components of other diseases. For example, "ague," once a disease in its own right, is now known as the cyclic fever of malaria. In Germany, physicians treat millions of patients for low blood pressure, a condition not even recognized as a disease in the United States. Remarkably, diseases can even appear or vanish by vote. During my own career, professional organizations put alcoholism on the disease list and took homosexuality off. There's been no ballot yet on a number of controversial conditions, including chronic fatigue syndrome, fibromyalgia, hypoglycemia, candida allergy, attention deficit disorder, and seasonal affective disorder. Offering no argument for or against any condition being a disease, I only suggest that science isn't our only arbiter of "fact."

Considering the extent of all conceivable knowledge of physical disease, we've gleaned only a fraction, and even that is shaky. Of the little we believe we do know, progress will ultimately reveal much of it to be useless or even false. Hardly any portion of today's medical practice resembles that of a hundred years ago, and a century from now our most advanced efforts will look to our descendants like cupping and bleeding look to us. The good news and the bad news are identical, then: we're doing our best. In what is now a famous speech, a medical school dean cautioned his graduating class, "I'm sorry, but a third of what we taught you is incorrect. The problem is that we don't know which third."

If it chagrins you to learn that disease isn't the constant we pretend it to be, then perhaps you'll take heart in the notion that illness isn't pixie dust: compared with disease, illness is as stable as Gibraltar. Time, place, and person may alter its face, but its body, suffering, varies little. Today's pain, fear, and rage are the same sensations Sophocles described. When we see someone wailing in the street, ripping her hair out and rending her dress, we might not know the details of her pain, but there's no doubt in our mind that she's suffering.

CHARACTERISTICS OF SUFFERING

Suffering has been around so long, we deserve to understand it better. If we did, we'd find it linked to healing in the same way that darkness complements light. The more we can learn of its characteristics, the more readily we'll see that one path to healing is through the center of suffering.

Let's examine some of its features:

- Suffering is a permanent property of humanhood.

- Unlike physical disease, suffering can't be fixed.

- Suffering is extraordinarily individual.

- Suffering isn't always necessarily tragic.

- Suffering is painful to experience.

Suffering is permanent, as native to humanity as our opposable thumb. Despite any conceivable medical progress, suffering is here to stay. If tomorrow afternoon we were to wipe out lupus, multiple sclerosis, and cancer, we'd of course be jubilant. Those who would have died would now survive into old age. But then they'd suffer the degenerative diseases they were previously too young to encounter.

Or let's consider an even more optimistic vision. Say, as Kurt Vonnegut proposed in a story, we obliterated all disease, and so enjoyed indefinite lifespans. Would we then achieve nirvana? Think about it. Will Rogers said of real estate, "They ain't makin' any more of it." The planet can hold only so many people, and when eight robust generations share a single apartment in a world of increasing scarcity, which will be the more likely domestic atmosphere, bliss or mayhem?

I mention suffering's persistence not for pessimism's sake, but actually to keep our mission in practical scope. When we set out to heal someone, we can't do so with the hope of annihilating suffering itself. We can only make our modest, local, and eminently feasible attempt.

Suffering can't be fixed. Disease and illness are different, but not in the way that apples and oranges are. The difference is *dimensional,* more like apples and wonder. Inhabiting the physical world, disease is physically addressable, so at least we can conceive of curing it. But since illness isn't tangible, we can't cure it any more than we can patch together smashed hopes or glue whole a broken promise. Suffering can be sensed, expressed, interpreted, hopefully learned from, and ultimately navigated through, but it can't possibly be fixed.

That suffering is unfixable doesn't mean it's untreatable, only that it requires treatment qualitatively different from what we'd apply to physical disease. And don't think of suffering's unfixability as a disadvantage. On the contrary, its subjective nature makes healing possible within *any* physical situation.

Suffering is exquisitely individual. No matter what our disease, our suffering is unique to us and to the moment. It may consist of hopelessness on Wednesday, dietary anxieties on Thursday, and a snit on the weekend over the way someone treated us Friday. In fact, the very discernment of the unique aspects of suffering is the beginning of its treatment.

My friend Steven was being treated for bladder cancer by means of local chemotherapy instilled through a urinary catheter. At a support group meeting, another member, Rick, who also had bladder cancer, asked Steven how he was doing.

"Dreadful."

"Dreadful? How so?"

Steven whined, "Who likes having a catheter jammed up their urethra?" Describing the procedure for other members, he compared the doctor to John Henry slamming through the mountain.

Rick winced. "Yeah, it was like that for me, too. How does it make you feel?"

"Well, sad, kind of. Helpless. Being done to."

"Whatcha gonna do about it?"

"Do about it?"

"Yeah, do about it."

"Like what? What did you do?"

"Oh, I just put the thing in myself."

Steven was dumbfounded. The possibility had never occurred to him.

The following week he reported, "I asked the doctor if I could insert the catheter myself. He said no, but when I told him I wouldn't continue treatment under present circumstances, he relented. He showed me how to do it, and I found I did it far more bearably."

Healing his illness allowed Steven to remain on the chemotherapy that treated his disease. Had he not discovered that what bothered him wasn't his cancer but his discomfort with catheterization, he wouldn't have done anything effective about it, and his course might have been less salubrious and certainly less pleasant. As it turned out, Steven felt the experience made him more powerful, more apt to assert control in future situations.

Bernadette, who suffered from congestive heart failure, attended a support group for people with various chronic diseases. When another member asked her, "What bothers you most about being sick?" she replied immediately, "I can't work."

She described the job she'd had to leave, processing insurance documents for a small firm.

As she spoke, she came to new realizations. "You know," she commented, looking surprised, "the work was pretty dull, to tell you the truth. What I really liked—what actually made every day for me—was that we began the morning with coffee and doughnuts. We just sat and gabbed for a half-hour. The boss was great that way. She knew happy employees were effective employees. It was wonderful, and I miss it so much . . ." She began to cry.

Other group members conspired during the following week and brought coffee and doughnuts to the next meeting. When Bernadette saw the treats, she cried again. Everyone cried. Then they laughed, ate, drank, and gabbed. This became the group's regular routine. A month later Bernadette said, "Yeah, I have congestive heart failure. But I could do this for a long time."

Suffering isn't necessarily entirely tragic. A serious disease is undeniably catastrophic, but that needn't be the whole truth. Since it certainly changes lives, it can sometimes ultimately change them for the better. I should caution you that this possibility isn't obvious to everyone and can even be offensive to the newly diagnosed, who don't need to hear then how their overwhelming misery may be a blessing in disguise. Still, over time, suffering can reveal itself as a hard-shelled fortune cookie, a difficult path that can actually lead toward a better life.

A possibly lethal disease captures our attention like nothing else. Once we get through the initial turmoil, maybe we can acknowledge what we found convenient to ignore earlier, our mortality. Our days were *always* numbered, but accepting that fact now might encourage us to pick and choose our moment-to-moment priorities. Once we're convinced we don't own time, only rent it from a merciless landlord, then we'll know that whatever we need to do in this life, we'd better get started.

Recognition of mortality, then, can be a gift as well as a tragedy. The realization that every sixty seconds of past is a minute less of future is a vitamin I wish I'd begun to take in the second grade. I'd even recommend it over fluoride in reservoirs. When I become more flamboyant, you'll find me distributing Certificates of Mortality door-to-door.

Life-threatening diseases can bear unexpected benefits, then, precisely because of their threat. Dozens of people have told me, "If it hadn't been for my lupus [or cancer, or kidney disease, or multiple sclerosis], I'd never have been able to leave that awful job [or return to painting, or forgive my children, or get my divorce, or take that trip]."

This was the case with my friend Ed. Without warning, Ed became drowsy and progressively unarousable at work. His colleagues called an ambulance. The hospital staff quickly diagnosed him as a new, insulin-dependent diabetic. They admitted him and with some difficulty stabilized him over the next few days.

Ed's supervisor visited and informed him that he'd be able to take at least a month's disability leave.

Ed's nurse Amanda asked him one morning what was on his mind.

"My disability leave," he answered.

"How so?"

"Strange, but I'm looking forward to it. I thought about going back to work, and I shuddered."

"What do you do?"

"Social work, with abusive families." He made a face. "I'm getting to hate it, frankly. I didn't realize that before. Being sick is like playing hockey and being sent to the penalty box; you can't play your little part, but you do get to watch the whole game. The game doesn't look so good to me now. I'm starting to wonder about going back. I don't have to, you know."

A year later, Ed said, "I found another job in the system. This doesn't upset me like my other one did. In fact, I'm having a much better time. I'm using my skills and accomplishing something worthwhile."

My friend Pat experienced something even more dramatic. Depressed for most of her adult life, she was usually medicated and had been hospitalized nine times. Then she developed breast cancer at the age of forty-five. As she recovered from her mastectomy, she was shocked to realize that her depression had inexplicably vanished. She became a highly energetic and effective breast cancer patient advocate. She confided to me, "This may sound a little crazy, but I wonder if maybe sometimes diseases are actually treatments for worse conditions."

Suffering is painful to experience. When we're sick, we're generally not eager to explore our suffering. After all, it hurts, and who wouldn't prefer pleasure? So I doubt that you'll like feeling your sick friend or relative's suffering any more than you'd be drawn to your own.

Yet there you are, riding along on hers. As your sense of her pain increases, you may understandably encounter times when you'll balk and want to get off the bus. You're feeling more than you can handle and so feel moved to stop the conversation. Ironically, you'll probably do it by offering her some kind of fix.

At her weekly bridge game, Madeleine, who felt well but who'd recently been diagnosed with pancreatic cancer, said, "Well, I've gone a little farther in figuring out what to do. I have an appointment next week with Dr. S., a surgeon. But I'm just not sure."

From Madeleine's right, Gladys immediately responded, "Dr. S.? Have you checked him out? I talked to my sister-in-law. She had surgery for the same thing, and she had Dr. N., who's the top one in the country, I hear."

From Madeleine's left, Minnie said, "Oh, I'd go to Johns Hopkins. I've been reading about the way they train surgeons there."

Finally Madeleine's bridge partner, Ruth, spoke. "Madeleine, you said you aren't sure. Aren't sure about what?"

"Well, I'm not sure I want to have surgery at all."

Now, why did Gladys and Minnie offer Madeleine their answers before knowing what her question was? From having done exactly the same thing numerous times, I believe I know. They sincerely wished to help her. Beneath that, they may have had more selfish motives, as we all occasionally do. Maybe they wanted to demonstrate how well informed or helpful they were.

But I suspect something even deeper, a purely emotional impetus: Madeleine's situation caused them pain. When the poet Virgil guided Dante through Hell in *The Divine Comedy*, he must have felt the heat, too. As companion to your sick friend or relative, sensing her suffering as she describes it, you'll suffer to some extent along with her. Such is the cost of compassion.

Madeleine's friends didn't like to see her in pain for her own sake, and further, hearing about her torment raised specters from their own past and present suffering, along with their worries about their future, to the point that they reached their limit. Their comments amounted to: I love you, but this is as far along your trail of tears as I can accompany you right now.

Their attempts to fix were simultaneously gambits to change the subject, end that particular conversation.

If you find yourself trying to fix your sick loved one, then, assume you're seeking to stop your own pain. That you're feeling her discomfort attests to your compassion, and that you want to relieve it attests to your humanhood. Later in the book I'll describe how you can address this snag, but for now, just be aware that it can happen.

SUFFERING AS A PATH TO HEALING

In suffering's core is the key to its release. As you might have noted in most of the stories in this chapter, suffering sensed finely enough reveals its own treatment. If you are to heal your sick friend or relative, begin by ignoring her disease and concentrating instead on her illness. Listen well, and she'll enter her suffering, explore it, know it, and unfold it for you. Listen even more deeply, and *she'll* comprehend her story and then act accordingly.

Bette, who'd had amyotrophic lateral sclerosis ("Lou Gehrig's disease") for several years, was rapidly declining. Only her husband, Keith, could understand her feeble whispers.

"I'm scared," she said.

Frightened himself by this statement, all Keith could think to say was "Tell me."

"I don't know," she said, and Keith sat silently. After a few minutes Bette continued. "I'm not scared of dying. I'm curious about it. But I'm scared I'll be so scared while I'm dying that I'll miss most of it. I don't want to go through it like that."

"Yeah," Keith replied. "You look scared now. But I know you better than anybody, and I don't think of you as fearful. We've been in situations where I've been afraid and you haven't. What's changed? What makes you think you'll be scared?"

Bette blinked a couple of times, meaning she'd spoken enough for now.

The following day she told Keith, "I took a deep look. If I haven't been scared till now, why would I think I'd ever be scared? I've gotten this far without fear. If I'm scared at the time, then I'm scared. That's the way it is. But now, I'm not."

Keith said, "Bette, scared or not scared, I'm so proud of you." He sat with her another thirty minutes, holding her hand. Late that night, Bette died in her sleep.

Revelations like Bette's don't await us congenially behind a "welcome" mat. On the contrary, even the ancients observed that they initially warn us away. The bulk of the Old Testament's Book of Job describes the poor man's fruitless attempts to understand and respond effectively to his afflictions. At last he throws himself on divine mercy. When God finally speaks to him, it isn't as a quiet aside, a pearl from a kindly uncle. No, God speaks from out of a whirlwind: that is, Job's healing begins when he squarely faces his suffering, however chaotic, however mysterious it first appears.

Pursue a healing conversation to its absolute end and you'll arrive at a mystery. By mystery I don't mean something unknowable, but rather puzzle pieces jumbled together. This apparent randomness is deceptive, for it's ultimately as precise a manifestation as a dream. Deep within your sick friend or relative, the naked elements of her suffering hint at its resolution. Her healing mystery is a question that contains its own answer. Well explored, her mystery will dissolve into a powerfully motivating truth.

I worked with Connie, who had a rare cancer of her endocrine system. Her doctors had removed her thyroid and adrenal glands and kept her on a strict regimen of replacement hormones. Middle-aged, single, and quite reserved, Connie lived alone, worked solo, had no close friends.

When a new, painless mass appeared in her abdomen, she came to me to clarify what she made of it.

"My doctor said the cancer's back," she said, "and he's doubtful much more can be done medically except to treat my symptoms. So I want to see what I might be able to do about it myself."

"What've you thought about it?" I asked.

"Well, actually, I've been keeping a diary. I wrote 'This feels like it's filling a void.' In fact, the void's catching my attention more than the mass is. What do you suppose the void is?"

"I don't know," I answered. "Sounds worth exploring, though."

Over the next week, Connie wrote about the void in her diary. She hadn't a clue to interpreting it, so she wrote instead about how she sensed it. She wrote that it was big, filling most of her body. It felt vacuumlike, too, as though it were imploding her, sucking her away from outside contact.

She told me, "I wrote all this stuff, and then I read it and reread it. It only confirms what I thought about myself. I've known for years that I resist relationships. But I'm beginning to realize I'm so lonely I could die, and have been for a long time. My sense of this mass is that it's filling the void in my life."

Connie decided to act on the hint, to seek authentic relationships. Of course, this was no small order. Reducing her aloofness amounted to changing her personality. But mortality can be a fine motivator. Over the next couple of months Connie became obviously warmer, approachable. The shift was dramatic, as though she'd metaphorically died and been reborn.

Now, three years later, she says, "I met Arthur, and we fell in love. At my age! That mass in my belly shrank, and I can't find it anymore. I haven't gone for checkups in a year now. I feel fine, and to tell you the truth, I'd rather pay attention to my life than worry about disease."

If Connie's abdominal mass was a cancer that regressed, then we can rejoice. But even if it had continued to grow and it finally took her life, we'd have had grounds to rejoice as well, for Connie emerged a markedly happier person for having consciously engaged her mystery. With or without a cure, she was definitively healed.

If you're to serve as a catalyst for transformations such as Connie's, how can we describe your role? You're not, after all, her doctor, and in any event this approach assiduously avoids her disease. Nor are you her psychotherapist. This isn't therapy: we assume her suffering's entirely normal; we don't assign her a diagnosis, recommend treatment, keep records, or bill anyone. The best description of your relationship is that you're her companion, possibly her guide. In sum, the endeavor seems most like plain old friendship.

One service that defines a close friend is listening well. If your sick loved one is to enter her whirlwind and retrieve her mystery, you must begin by encouraging her to express her feelings. She'll speak to the extent she trusts you're listening. To listen with the requisite intensity, you'll need to stop whatever else you're doing and become extraordinarily quiet.

TO HEAL

1. Focus on the sick person's feelings. Recognizing that she's suffering not from her disease but from her emotional experience of it, focus on her emotional

(continued)

responses. If she comments, "They're going to do that blood test tomorrow," you can ask, "How do you feel about the test?" ⚬

2. Invite her to speak to you about her feelings, but don't pressure her. At first, when she may be too devastated even to speak, you can help simply by being with her. You can say, "It's all right that you don't want to talk about it now. Would you like to be alone, or would you like me to just sit with you?" ⚬

3. If she's anxious about what she's feeling, assure her that whatever she feels is normal. The emotions that she experiences are a normal feature of her sickness and will pass with time. You can say, "It's obvious you're having a hard time now. That's part of being sick. The only way to get through it is by getting through it, and I'll be with you all the way." ⚬

4. Keep your own speech to a minimum. Her healing will emerge mainly from her own statements. As you listen to her, expect that her suffering will be unique to her, may hold unexpected benefits, and may cause *you* pain. ⚬

THREE

BEING PRESENT

> *Healing requires that you give your full,*
> *unconditional, loving attention to the sick person.*

We can make our minds so like still water that beings gather about
us to see their own images, and so live for a moment with a clearer,
perhaps even with a fiercer life because of our silence.

—William Butler Yeats

Through love, all pain is turned to medicine.

—Rumi

HEALING REQUIRES YOUR PROFOUND PRESENCE

When I was six, I tripped playing in the street one afternoon,
skinned my knee, and ran home howling. I'll bet you suffered a
similar tragedy at that age, and that your mother treated your
wound like my mother treated mine. She poured stinging orange
liquid on it, dabbed it dry, and applied a Band-Aid. That was
her medical technology, her treatment to cure my injury. Then,

by holding me and kissing my boo-boo, she healed me: my fear and pain evaporated.

Our mothers knew kissing us wouldn't erase our scrapes, that cures would come with time. As for healing us, they never questioned whether kissing boo-boos was scientific or whether they were qualified to treat us. Kids heal because of the intense connection between them and their parents.

Healing is about kissing boo-boos.

We comfort people best when we contact them closely. How closely can we contact them? Cole Porter asked that question in his 1930 song "The Physician":

Once I loved such a shattering physician,
Quite the best-looking doctor in the state.
He looked after my physical condition,
And his bedside manner was great.

When I'd gaze up and see him there above me,
Looking less like a doctor than a Turk,
I was tempted to whisper, "Do you love me,
Or do you merely love your work?"

He said my bronchial tubes were entrancing.
My epiglottis filled him with glee.
He simply loved my larynx and went wild about
    my pharynx,
But he never said he loved me . . .

He admired my physical parts, but what about the rest of me? Of course, Porter was hinting as usual at romance, but his song also speaks of our craving for love in our illness, someone to kiss our boo-boo. Who should that someone be? Whose responsibility is it to love sick people, and what do we mean by love, anyway?

Whether or not doctors should love their patients, you as a caregiver certainly have the opportunity. You'll be with your sick friend or relative through crucial, possibly agonizing experiences. Like buddies in a foxhole, you'll forge an emotional bond. You can refine the bond into a healing relationship that intensifies his trust, helps him access deeper feelings, and supports his own therapeutic efforts.

THE CENTER OF HEALING IS LOVE

I call the bond that develops between you and your sick friend or relative *love*. If that word raises your hackles, welcome to the club. I'm tempted to avoid it, appalled as I am by its loose and often manipulative usage. Depending on the speaker's intent, love can mean attraction, reverence, friendship, sex, romance, or lust.

When I speak about healing, though, I find I must use it—after taking pains to explain what I mean by it. By love I mean *attention*. Loving your sick friend or relative means giving him your complete presence, nothing more or less. Questions of liking or disliking, of desire, repulsion, flirtation, or rejection are, for healing purposes, irrelevant to loving him.

Attention may strike you as an unorthodox way of envisioning love. But it fills our bill, so I'll stand by it. When my mother kissed my wound, she wasn't adoring me but simply being with me thoroughly. Aware I was literally in her care, my fear and trembling disappeared, however ragged my knee.

When we're sick, we yearn for something similar from those who attend us. At the least, we require practitioners to be technically competent; their caring presence is a fine bonus. We don't ask them to court us—though it's always nice when they like us—only genuinely to be with us and not just in physical proximity.

I don't think it's possible to overrate sick people's need for attention. A few years ago, a university medical center surveyed its former patients about their experiences when hospitalized. One question was, "Of all personnel, which helped you most to feel better?" Response categories included physicians, nurses, and technicians, but the runaway winner was a write-in, housekeepers.

Who's the housekeeper? She's the lady with the aching back who wheels her mop bucket into your room in the quiet hours and asks, "How're you doing?" She probably hasn't a notion of the condition of your intestines and coronaries. She's there to clean the floor, but she needs to rest a bit first and would love a little company.

That is, patients say they get their best emotional help from people who are interested in *them*, not particularly in their disease. Actually, I suspect this research may be apocryphal, but it captured my fancy because people in cancer support groups have been telling me similar versions for years. When we feel recognized, witnessed, understood, we shine. We feel tangibly better: recognition is a major healing stimulant, on a par, I'd say, with adequate sleep.

If closeness promotes healing, then we're asking for trouble when we increase distance. As much as sick people love being heard, they get angry when they're not heard. Some colleagues and I recently asked a number of cancer patients extensive questions about their entire medical experience. As we expected, they offered both positive and negative comments. The latter fell almost entirely into one area, not being noticed or heard or appreciated—that is, not being loved. They told tale after tale of healthcare practitioners, friends, and family members failing to take their feelings or opinions seriously, as though their sickness had rendered them transparent, canceled their personhood. Not only was their suffering unrelieved, but they were angry, sometimes to the point of litigation. In fact, medical malpractice attorneys have known for decades that most suits don't come from medical mayhem, but from poor doctor-patient relationships.

PROTECTING OURSELVES FROM OTHERS' SUFFERING

If my message were only "Love sick people and they'll heal," I would've written a bumper sticker instead of a book. The real world isn't that simple. Even when we're convinced that intimacy heals, we tend to hold ourselves back. We understandably ask, Won't the suffering of others overwhelm me? Won't it flood my emotions and drive me toward "burnout"? This issue is so reasonable and so universal, I'm not about to minimize it. It can't but be on the mind of anyone who engages in healing.

As you ponder this quandary, you'll no doubt seek models, people who work regularly with suffering. Of course, the most accessible models are healthcare professionals. You'll find that they protect themselves by generally maintaining some emotional distance from sick people. It's not an explicit course in their training, but doctors and nurses learn that if they involve themselves emotionally with a sick person, they'll lose precious objectivity and, in addition, stagger toward exhaustion.

Strangely, while this view makes sense, I've found no scientific evidence to support it. The healing relationship being my field of interest, I read all I can about it, and I have never found substantiation that a close connection jeopardizes either party. On the contrary, I have found research suggesting that intimacy, once it's acknowledged, can heal both.

Even those who opt to create emotional distance can't achieve more than a pretense of it. I defy those whose hands and fingers daily explore *inside* other people to tell me with a straight face that they aren't involved with them. When we're immersed in people's feelings, we can't help but be influenced by them. So if you're concerned about emotional overload, you should know you won't burn out from being present to the suffering of others but from your efforts to ignore and repress the suffering you've already absorbed.

I suspect that at the bottom of this issue is our wish to avoid the pain of loving people who will die. A death hurts to the degree we're close to the decedent. Yet everyone dies. I was initially shocked to realize I'll lose everyone I love: I'll die first or they will. There's no choice in this, but there is choice in how I wish to spend my time with them. If my prime desire is to protect myself from hurting, I'll minimize intimacy. But that protection comes at a mortal cost, the very juice of life. That is, love and suffering can't be separated.

Compassion literally means "suffer with," so when you feel what the sick person feels, you'll hurt. Your pain doesn't mean you're being physically damaged; it's only a feeling that washes through you. Yet because we are culturally conditioned to avoid pain, your first reaction may be to back away, decline to hear more. A few years ago, as I prepared to speak to a large group of physicians about the healing relationship, I was chatting with the internist who was to introduce me.

"Exactly what's your practice?" he asked.

"Basically, I listen to patients."

"Hey, that's what I do. I spend almost all my time talking to my patients."

I didn't comment on his choice of words. He asked me to jot down a few autobiographical notes for him, so I wrote what I'd mentioned, that I listen to patients.

Introducing me later, he read directly from my note: ". . . Dr. Kane's practice is mainly talking to patients . . ."

Use it or lose it: close your ears long enough, and they'll seal over. If you find yourself withdrawing emotionally, simply recognize you're doing it, appreciate it as understandable, and forgive yourself. Then admit a little more suffering into your sensibility in each ensuing encounter. In this way you'll progress toward greater healing, perhaps for the sick person but certainly for yourself.

HEALING WITH FULL ATTENTION

Your presence is a fundamental requirement for healing. In fact, sometimes it's sufficient in itself. Be there, sense what's happening, and then let events take their course.

My friend Cary, who'd battled lung cancer for years, had his quarterly checkup. "My doctor phoned me and asked me to come in. He'd always given me results by phone, so I suspected the worst. When I saw him, that's what I got. He told me my tumors had spread, and there was nothing more he could do medically except relieve my symptoms.

"When I got home from that visit, I sank into the sofa and told my wife, Helen. I didn't expect her to do something magic and cure me, but I also didn't expect her to do what she did. I remember this clearly, as though it happened in slow motion. A tear formed in Helen's eye and ran down her cheek. She didn't say a word, just showed me what she felt, which was exactly what

I felt. I realized that was all I really wanted, for her to be there with me. She didn't have to do anything else."

Sometimes sick people need only to know that someone has honestly witnessed their suffering. Helen was able to do that thoroughly for Cary because none of her attention leaked elsewhere.

Considering how we normally operate, full attention is quite an order. In our daily world we tend to listen with a partial ear, observe with a restless eye. However much we may claim full presence, it's likely that a three-ring circus is cavorting on our mental stage. Sure, I'm listening to you, I say, but the truth is that I'm attending as well to my neck pain, my retirement benefits, fantasies about that person just past your shoulder, and, not least, my anxieties about your condition. I can barely follow my own pageant, let alone yours. Gestalt therapy originator Fritz Perls advised those of us mesmerized blind by our mind-play, "Lose your mind and come to your senses."

STOP

Our standard social pace may help us lose our minds, albeit in a perverse way, but we'll come to our senses only when we stop. Obviously, I can't commune deeply while I'm chafing to escape to my next appointment. If I'm to help a sick person understand his present situation, we both need to attend to what is here, now—and that means stopping.

Author Milan Kundera, in his intriguing novel *Slowness,* contrasts our current concept of pace with that of two hundred years ago, when communication technology's cutting edge was a handwritten note delivered by a servant on horseback. If the luxury of the space age is speed, that of our ancestors was continuity. Writes Kundera:

There is a secret bond between slowness and memory, between speed and forgetting. Consider this utterly commonplace situation: a man is walking down the street. At a certain moment, he tries to recall something, but the recollection escapes him. Automatically, he slows down. Meanwhile, a person who wants to forget a disagreeable incident he has just lived through starts unconsciously to speed up his pace, as if he were trying to distance himself from a thing still too close to him in time.

Relentless motion separates us from the context of our lives. When we deliberately stop, our trailing historical wake catches up to us. Our senses shift: no longer having to strain to see where we're going, we can relax and see where we are. So don't just do something, sit there.

In 1928 Dr. Alexander Fleming demonstrated how valuable this simple skill can be. He didn't set out to discover penicillin, only to study a particular bacterium. One Friday afternoon, one of his technicians mistakenly left the covers off several culture plates. When Fleming returned Monday morning, he found the bacterial colonies on those plates destroyed, apparently by a mold spore that had floated in through his window from a laboratory downstairs. His experiment ruined, Fleming had every right to bellow rage. But he was an authentic scientist, so he let go of his abstract goal for the moment, considered instead what was before his eyes, and in doing so earned a Nobel Prize and knighthood.

The pace of the healing encounter is slower than that of a social encounter. Expect periods of apparent inactivity and silence. I say "apparent" because when people stop speaking, it's not necessarily because their brains went cold. On the contrary, they're likely thinking, perhaps assembling some thought they've never before expressed.

The Skill of Silence

To heal, stop and then get quiet. Silence brings focus. Just as we can fill a cup to the extent we've first emptied it, we can hear a sick person to the extent we've quieted our mind. How quiet do we need to get? Some cultures have raised silence to an art form. Zen Buddhists learn as they sit still to transform their attention to an all-receptive void. Christian monastics contemplate for months at a time, sinking endlessly into their subject. Yogis can so quiet themselves that their pulse and respiration fall to the barely viable, where they experience sensation undecorated by thought. Compared to these Olympian feats, our task seems rudimentary. I'm not asking anyone to sit on a Himalayan ledge, only to stop all else and quietly attend a sick friend or relative. You can get to this point by downshifting from a preoccupied high gear to a more attentive neutral: the motor's running, but you're not going anywhere at the moment.

Your silence doesn't precede the "real" work; it pervades it just as a tune necessarily blends its notes with the spaces between them.

I learned this from a carpenter friend. A few years ago when I hired Bram to build a deck, he warned me to expect something novel. "It's Japanese joinery," he cautioned. "It's not like carpentry here. Sometimes it'll look like I'm not working."

"Fine," I agreed, captured as usual by exotica.

Bram arrived on the appointed morning, sat on his toolbox, and stared at the space that would be the deck. I was paying him by the hour, so after he'd stared most of the morning, I began to question my judgment. Finally Bram stood up, dusted off, and said, "Okay."

Then he sharpened his chisels for an hour.

As Bram passed his blades over flat stones, leather, and finally rice paper, he offered me gems of samurai sharpening lore. I hadn't known that at night a proper edge reflects the North Star.

At noon he lined up his tools, took a full breath, said, "There," and went into action. Wood flew, joined, locked in place. The deck steadily appeared, less as an earthly structure than as a poem written elegantly into its place.

Bram accomplished something as extraordinary as it is, well, ordinary: he did one thing at a time. He planned, then he sharpened his tools, and then he built. Focusing exclusively on the work at hand, he discharged each task thoroughly. Whether we build a deck, bake a pie, or sit with a sick person, we'll perform exactly as well as we can focus. The quality of your healing work will depend on your single-minded presence, your ability to quiet yourself, to be receptive rather than expressive.

MINIMIZE YOUR WORDS AND BODY LANGUAGE

It's not enough to avoid speaking, though that's a decent start. Even when we don't speak, we normally maintain a level of physical and mental activity that for healing purposes is superfluous. So in order to listen, we don't speak, of course, but we don't move, either. And beyond that, we don't even think.

Not speaking means expressing neither words nor body language. We often indicate we're listening by nodding and commenting. "Oh, yes," we respond. "Uh-huh." But nodding and commenting are expressions, and when we express anything, we're not listening. In addition, our responses to the sick person, sparse though they may be, will encourage him here, inhibit him there—that is, influence his direction and contaminate his story. Believe me, when we purely listen, it's obvious. We don't have to announce we're doing it. Most of us can manage this level of silence.

STOP YOUR MENTAL CHATTER

In healing mode, we don't think. Plainly, this is a greater test. After all, we've thought all our lives. Thinking is what the mind does for a living. It actually doesn't know how to do anything else, so when we ask it to take even a short break, it objects as though we'd threatened its very life. It's so cunning in its insistence on staying active that it's known in Hindu lore as the drunken monkey. One of the mind's myriad ploys might be to persuade us that it and we are one and the same, that if we turned it off even for a moment, we'd die.

But all that happens when we stop thinking is that we suspend our habitual way of understanding the world, including any notions about the sick person we're with. When we view him from our own inner quiet, absent our customary interpretations, we'll see him a little differently. In particular, we'll be very much with him instead of with our ideas about him, which is to say, with ourselves.

The mind is hard to quiet partly because it's such a subtle function. Normally, it chatters incessantly, buzzes so constantly that we don't recognize it any more than a fish recognizes water. Failing to notice it, we can easily believe ourselves silent when we're actually in mental riot. The task, then, isn't to get quiet as much as to learn what quiet *is*. The most effective, time-honored, accessible technology I know for doing so is meditation. If you don't already meditate, read about it, ask friends who do meditate, and try the exercise I'll offer below.

That grain of suggestion comes with a bushel of gentle caution: in learning to meditate, please be patient with yourself. Why is it we'd forgive ourselves if we couldn't stand up right now and do ten pull-ups, but we whip ourselves silly when we fail to achieve grade-A meditation on our first try? We assume it must be easy since by definition it's doing nothing at all. Quieting the mind, though, is actually a lot like doing pull-ups: it's arduous and frustrating, *and* proficiency grows with practice. I saw a cartoon in which a wise old monk advises a circle of novices, "Enlightenment is a long process that requires diligence and patience. That's why I asked you to bring sandwiches."

As you gain silence, your sick friend or relative will of course appreciate your presence, but you yourself will enjoy a curious side-benefit: your increased presence makes you less distractible in other situations. This will be especially useful when occasionally relatives or even healthcare practitioners swirl frantically around you and the sick person. Their hyperactivity may be appropriate, but if you're not prepared, its intensity can corrupt your silence and even call into question the value of your healing efforts. Adequately established presence will stabilize you in such a storm and may even recenter those around you. In his poem "If," Rudyard Kipling emphasized the importance of remaining focused within chaos:

If you can keep your head when all about you
Are losing theirs and blaming it on you . . .
[then] yours is the Earth and everything that's in it . . .

My friend Rachel was primary caregiver for her eighty-two-year-old mother, Sophie. Rachel's frustration mounted as her mother's needs increased, and soon she began to suffer anxiety and insomnia. She joined a meditation class to try to deal with these symptoms and, indeed, over the next few weeks noticed more mental peace as well as increased physical stamina.

Sophie declined rapidly, though. Her doctor hospitalized her for severe, progressive heart disease. When at last her brain's oxygen supply fell below the critical level, she went into a coma. Rachel summoned her brother and two sisters from other states.

Once at their mother's bedside, they began to express their preferences for Sophie's treatment. The sisters demanded that everything possible be done to keep her alive, that she be maintained artificially at all costs. The brother, aghast at this prospect, insisted that medical assistance be immediately withdrawn and Sophie be allowed to die. The argument re-opened ancient grudges, and soon they were screaming at one another.

Rachel, however, said not a word, only sat. She quietly held her mother's hand while practicing her meditation skills. When finally her siblings paused for breath, Rachel said, "Excuse me, but can you back off the past and future for a couple of min-utes and pay attention to what's happening right now?"

This caught their attention. They stopped arguing and sat thoughtfully the rest of the afternoon. Later that evening, they were able to discuss their feelings and reach compromises that Rachel, as Sophie's named legal agent, effected.

Perhaps you have no experience with meditation, so I'll offer you an exercise as a preview. Don't think of meditation as any-thing more than deep relaxation. It's best if you can record the exercise on tape and then play it back to yourself as a guide.

While you record, speak more slowly than you ordinarily would. Since the tape instructs you in certain exercises, you'll need time to perform each, so leave gaps between sentences. Your complete recording should span about ten minutes.

Recordable Relaxation/Meditation Exercise

First, allow yourself time and space for getting quiet. Unplug your phone; there's no message that can't wait ten minutes. Close doors so you have privacy, and ask those with whom you live not to interrupt you.

Now sit as you would at a bedside, attending above all else to your comfort. Balance yourself so you're neither straining to be upright nor likely to fall over as you deeply relax.

Do nothing now except to notice how your body feels at this moment. Don't fight yourself or curse yourself if you fidget, twitch, or itch. Give in to these distractions to your heart's content, and they'll go their way.

Now you're sitting quietly, without moving. Explore this stillness in your body. Don't comment on it; simply feel where you're at rest.

Notice your breath. It flows in and out, rises and falls like a tide. How peaceful can your breath become? Begin to imagine yourself breathing passively, as though the breath comes and goes on its own, without your work. Pretend that instead of you having to draw sustenance from the universe, the universe is benevolently supplying you with no effort on your part. All you need to do is get out of the way, let the breath simply happen.

Now sense what your feet feel like. Feel the peace, the absence of movement or tension.

If you can sense your feet easily, good. But your mind may rebel at this bid for silence, so that your attention, instead of going to your feet, goes to an old memory or your next meal or some noise on the street. Like an unruly child, the mind wants to wander. It's all right if it distracts you. There's nothing wrong with you. On the contrary, your mind is functioning normally.

But it's your tool, not the other way around, so it needs some gentle training. Every time you notice a distraction, return your attention to your passive respiration, the feel of your breath flowing in and flowing out. Let your body breathe in its most natural style, whatever that is for you. In all this exercise, don't change your natural breath. All you're changing is the way you *notice* your breath.

Now bring your attention to your calf muscles. Notice their passive softness, and notice how your knees feel while they're not bearing weight.

Sense your thighs, your upper legs. They're loose, not needing to be tight or to move.

Sense your pelvis. If you notice any tight muscles, release them. If you're unsure whether a muscle is tight, then deliberately tighten it, so you know, and then you can let it go.

How soft can your belly be? With each breath cycle, pretend you're directing your inspiration into your belly, so that its skin bulges outward. With expiration, that skin falls back softly, toward the front of your spine.

Now feel how your ribs move with your breath. Feel how they rise slightly and expand to the sides when you breathe in, and fall when you breathe out. Pretend the air you've breathed in is massaging the inside of your chest wall, softening the small muscles between your ribs.

Sense your neck and your throat. Notice that when you inhale, your windpipe widens slightly.

If you feel any tension anywhere, pretend to direct a breath into that area, and let the breath soften it.

Feel your shoulders, arms, wrists, and hands. There's nothing happening there now. What does that feel like?

Again, if your mind wants to tug you away from this exercise, simply notice that, thank it for its cleverness, and return your attention to your passive breath. You may notice yourself becoming sleepy, drifting off and thinking this would be a great opportunity for a nap. That thought is another of your mind's distractions. Come back to your breath. Each time.

Now bring your attention to your face. You're relaxing, so you don't need to use a single facial muscle. Imagine in your mind's eye that you're seeing your face. Is there any expression, however slight? If so, soften it so your face shows only deep relaxation.

Your entire body is now maximally at peace. What does this feel like? How much of your relaxed body can you sense at once? That isn't easy, so be patient with yourself if you don't feel your whole body at once. It's all right to *pretend*, to imagine what your peaceful body might feel like.

In any case, feel what you feel without internally commenting on it. You're now at this session's maximum point of relaxation. Feel it now without words over the next thirty seconds.

[*Leave a thirty-second silence on the tape.*]

To the extent you can feel this degree of relaxation, your body memorizes it, making it easier to repeat at will in the future.

Over the next couple of breath cycles, allow your eyes to open gently. You may notice resistance to this, since it feels so peaceful with your eyes closed. Regard that resistance as distraction, though, and let your eyes open anyway. Once they're open, let them behave as they will. They may focus; they may not. They may blink and wander.

It's a little more difficult to feel relaxed once your eyes are open, even though they're soft. It seems you're more in the physical world, with its attractions and demands. But continue to stay with your breath. You're secure in your inner world now, and peaceful in your outer world. Feel what this feels like, to be at peace in your body and in the world. Here's what this sensation is called: normal.

Now give your mind permission to think again. Before you return to your daily life, congratulate yourself for whatever degree of silence you sensed, no matter how small or fleeting it seemed to you. This skill is a difficult one, and you're on your way.

SEE THE WHOLE PERSON, NOT JUST HIS SICK ASPECT

Even when we're not thinking, we might still carry subtle cultural attitudes that flavor our perceptions about the sick person and our relationship with him. One of these attitudes is that he's a "patient," and another is that we're there to "heal" him.

Since full attention, healing love, is by definition unconditional, these attitudes will impede healing. We need to accept the sick person cleanly, without applying judgments about his physical condition, his prognosis, our contact with him, or its outcome.

Muriel, in remission from colon cancer, described a phenomenon "patients" commonly experience. "Holy Toledo!" she exclaimed. "It's like I've got a big *C* branded on my forehead and nine toes in the grave! I'm sure that's why the people I work with are all hugs and honey these days. The woman in the next cubicle, who for the past twenty-two years has greeted me with 'How are you?' now looms up to me nose-to-nose, and it's 'How aaaaaare you?' Mr. Personnel catches me in the hall and squirms, 'Um, we didn't invite you to the company picnic because, ah, we thought you might be, ah, sick.' My friend Ingrid looks me up and down like she's measuring me for a casket and marvels, 'You don't look like you have cancer.' My niece Charlene, even. We're having dinner at her place. I finish and stand up with my plate, and it's, 'Muriel, you sit down. I don't want you to wash a single dish.'

"I know they mean well. But I wouldn't say they make me feel better. In fact, I come away from those scenes believing I'm sicker than I thought, and lonelier, for sure."

In ways both crude and subtle, we generally regard sick people as less than those who aren't sick: less robust, of course, but also less competent, less proactive, and even less physically present. Consider the many little elements in standard medical practice that encourage the patient to feel diminished and relatively helpless. He too often waits endlessly, patiently, so to speak, for the doctor. Then he undresses and lies passively on the examining table while the doctor speaks a mysterious language and operates incomprehensible machinery. How can someone not feel intimidated?

This phenomenon isn't just medical; it's fully cultural. We complain of our symptoms with words of moral weight: there's something "wrong" with us, we "feel bad," "feel like hell." When we miss work and others need to fill in for us, we feel unproductive, that we let people down. It isn't good to be sick. I'm sure our popular notion that medicine must hurt to be effective descends from the medieval practice of beating the devil out of the sick.

To the extent we see the sick person as a "patient" we'll relate to his patienthood instead of his wider identity. In particular, we'll undervalue his strengths. While he's sick, remember, he's unusually vulnerable to the opinions of others, so if we see him as a helpless victim, he's likely to see himself that way, too. But if all parties can see the sickness principally as a *significant event*, which it unarguably is, he'll be in a better position to access all his resources.

That "patient" frame isn't an easy one to put down. Almost a quarter-century ago, a team of researchers learned how sticky that label can be. They recruited a number of volunteers from the general functioning population and had them present themselves at a variety of psychiatric hospitals. There they were to behave normally but confide to the admitting physician, "I feel like wood." (The researchers chose that particular phrase because it appears nowhere in psychiatric literature.) They were further instructed that if they were admitted, they were to inconspicuously keep a journal of their experiences.

All subjects were admitted. Once they were hospitalized, the psychiatric personnel saw them as abnormal even when bona fide patients objected that these new people obviously weren't crazy. The "pseudopatients" soon discovered that they could record their experiences openly. No one bothered to read what they wrote, since it was presumed to be psychotic gibberish. Having observed one subject working on his journal, a nurse recorded on his chart, "Exhibits writing behavior." Indeed, so fixed was the staff's delusion that the researchers sometimes had to go to extraordinary lengths to get their subjects discharged.[1]

You've probably read of similar studies: for example, teachers who've been told that a particular group of students is gifted grade them highly, while other teachers, informed that the same group is learning-disabled, grade them lower.

When we see someone we perceive as different from us—someone who's sick or disabled, say—we tend mentally to underline that difference, and sometimes even express it overtly. I have a middle-aged friend who's been in a wheelchair since his teens because of polio. He complains that regularly, when he's in a restaurant with his wife, the server takes her order and then asks her, "What'll *he* have?"

Sometimes we'll distance ourselves because of our feelings about a particular disease. Cancer still carries a degree of social stigma, and some people feel strongly about other diseases as well. Ten years ago, a member of a cancer support group asked, "Is this group open to people who have Kaposi's sarcoma?"

"What's that?" another member asked.

"It's a rare kind of cancer you can get when you have AIDS."

With that, three people arose and left without a word. I phoned each that night, asking what had happened. None would discuss their departure in the least, and they never attended another meeting.

Once we recognize some of the many associations the word *patient* can hold for us, how can we avoid placing a partition between ourselves and the sick person? How can we accept his undeniable physical situation without diminishing his personhood?

Fortunately, we already know how: familiarity. Discomfort with difference fades with steady contact. Years ago, I worked in an agency for disabled people alongside Francis, a professional counselor who'd been born with multiple deformities. When I first met him, his appearance made me gasp involuntarily. Francis heard me and went back to work: he'd heard it before. Over months, as I came to know him, externals wore off and I felt as comfortable with him as with anyone else. I presume he made similar progress in regard to any gasping he'd done about my appearance.

One morning, as he and I sat in his empty waiting room planning a conference, the automatic main door creaked open and a man in a wheelchair rolled in. A quadriplegic, he operated his motorized chair by means of a pointer strapped to his head. Sneering, Francis whispered to me, "Oh, my God. Here comes a drooler. I can't stand droolers."

Yet Francis might soon be one, and so might I. It was sobering, as one of a minority of nondisabled people in the agency, to be referred to as "our temporarily able-bodied friend." Physical differences are shallow and transitory. Genuine contact is that which occurs beyond body, color, gender, age, and infirmity. At that level, given your sick friend or relative's particular circumstances, he's normal, whole, and coping.

My friend Collin is a manufacturer who lost the use of one arm from a stroke and keeps it in a sling against his belly. I was with him one morning as he led a tour of children through his factory. A seven-year-old boy sidled up to Collin and asked, "Hey, what's wrong with your arm?"

Collin didn't bat an eye. "Nothing's wrong," he answered, "it just don't work."

"Oh," the boy grinned, "cool," and rejoined his group.

There are any number of ways to comprehend sickness. It can be an all-out catastrophe, a sacred test, a cross to bear, a painful lesson, divine vengeance, a meaningless physiological derangement, and so on. In the same way, the sick person can be a victim, a doomed wretch, a martyr, one of the chosen, and who knows what else. If we harbor no preconceptions, we're free to hear virtually any interpretation he cares to make. Sitting with him as we do, we can help him see himself in the most healing light.

One afternoon my friend Evan visited his support group connected, as usual, to his oxygen cylinder. When it was his turn to speak, he hesitated, looking embarrassed.

"I'm really ashamed of this," he said, "but I feel I can say anything here, so I'd like to just get it out. I didn't come last Wednesday because I was totally exhausted. My wife was working out of town then, so I was by myself. I got up one morning and became so short of breath getting dressed, I had to fall back into bed.

"I couldn't get up. I lay there and cried. Then I screamed. I was so angry. I couldn't do anything if I couldn't get up. Couldn't visit friends, go out anywhere. I even got breathless talking on the phone.

"I yelled 'I'm going to show you!' and I stayed right there and refused to eat or drink."

A group member asked, "Who were you yelling at, Evan, God?"

"I don't know if I believe in God. I was yelling at whatever was making me so damn weak, maybe the cancer. I stayed in bed two days and nights without eating. Oh, I made it to the bathroom once and I had a couple of sips of water."

"Why did you do that?"

"Yeah, why? Who knows why? When my wife finally came home, she found me in a state, let me tell you. I've never seen her so alarmed. She said I was trying to kill myself and began to force food into me. I don't think I meant to kill myself, but I see how she thought so. I feel really guilty now, ashamed of what I tried to do to myself and to her." Evan looked down into his lap.

"Wait a minute," someone said. "You think you were suicidal?"

"Sure. Wasn't I?"

"You don't sound to me like you were even depressed. You were angry, right?"

"Goddamn right I was angry! Wouldn't you be?"

"Sure would," said someone else. "I don't think you were suicidal, though. You were defiant. It was like those prison hunger strikers you hear about. When there's nothing else you can do, you can always refuse to eat. Maybe you were fighting back, doing what you could, like a warrior."

Evan stopped, stared straight ahead. "You think so?"

"Try it on."

"Gee," Evan laughed. "Yeah. Honestly, I never did mean to kill myself. I was plain furious. Maybe I was rebelling. Hah! Wait'll I tell my wife I wasn't suicidal; I was a warrior." He paused. "You really think so?"

"Well, whatever you did gave you energy. You made it here today."

Let Go of the Notion You'll Heal Anyone

The other major condition, or supposition, that can restrict your attention is that you are to "heal" the sick person. But wait, you say: how can you heal him unless you intend to?

Healing is a process, not a goal. It's all voyage and no destination. Your task is only to be present to the sick person. The moment you begin contemplating the encounter's outcome—whether he'll attain serenity or not, whether you'll "succeed" or "fail"—you're no longer with him but wandering in your own mind, oriented toward the future rather than the present. All you can ever do is your best; what is to be is out of your hands.

Mark Healing Time as Special

As you progress into healing work, don't devalue your regular daily life. Honor your interests outside healing, interests that validly demand your working, chattering mind. It's all right to converse with your sick friend or relative about the Atlanta Braves, curse the drought together, recall a memorable meal. Every encounter needn't be a karmic expedition.

If you maintain this distinction, you'll treat healing time as special. In fact, I even suggest you declare it as such. I've learned from effective healers to ritually mark the beginning and end of an encounter. For example, when I facilitate a cancer support group I ask that we observe a short silence as we begin. This way we slow to a halt and begin to focus on what's here rather than what isn't. In addition, we signify we've left the mundane world outside and entered one more dedicated to honesty, acceptance, and depth. At the end of the meeting I ask for a joining of hands around our circle, a sign that we're engaged, unified, secure, and complete.

Whether you use ritual markers or not, begin a session with an individual by first ensuring physical silence. Unplug the phone, close the door, and ask those outside the room to guard your privacy. Then, as a ritual of beginning, you can do what our groups do—simply sit quietly together for a minute. I know a woman who begins her individual sessions by deploying an altar she brings with her. Another rings a vibrant Tibetan bell. To mark the closing of an individual session, I request another minute of silence. I know others who close with hand-holding or hugs, and one who recites the Lord's Prayer. If you decide to use rituals, it's important that both parties be comfortable with them.

Practice your growing ability to become quieter with people who aren't sick. That is, refine your skill by getting deliberately quiet when, you might say, it doesn't count. At the next party you attend, listen to a new acquaintance as fully as you'd attend the sick. If you do that, you might notice that the healing relationship resembles nothing as much as plain old friendship, which happens to be the most healing of human contacts.

So stop, sit still, and clear your mind. As your friend or relative tells you about his illness, you'll find there's more than enough to occupy your complete presence.

TO HEAL

1. Quiet your mind before you join the sick person. Do so by means of the exercise in this chapter or some other discipline.

2. Make your time together extraordinary. Ensure privacy and quiet: close doors, unplug phones, prohibit intrusions. Consider marking the beginning and end of your meeting with a simple ritual.

3. Attend to him fully. Minimize your own words and body language in order to give him your full attention. When you do so, he'll sense it and consequently trust you more. His expression to you will be exactly as deep as his trust in you.

4. See him as the whole person he is. Sickness is only a part of his current experience. By honoring his talents and strengths as well, you'll remind him that those tools are available to him.

5. Let go of the notion that you'll heal him. Do your best without getting attached to the outcome. Stop thinking about whether he'll recover or die, whether you'll be of help, and what you believe he needs. Just be with him, now.

FOUR

LISTENING FOR
MEANING

> *If you listen skillfully to people's illness stories,*
> *they'll tell you how they can heal.*

Hope is not the conviction that something will turn out well, but the certainty that something makes sense regardless of how it turns out.
— Václav Havel, president, Czech Republic

I have to sing it my way. I don't know any other way.
— Billie Holiday

WE RESPOND TO ILLNESS ACCORDING TO
ITS MEANING

Two friends of mine, Hank and Thomas, had heart attacks a year ago.

Hank had long expected his. "My father and uncle both died of heart attacks," he says. "My older brother had one when he was the age I am now. I guess it comes with the territory for the males in our family."

After he left the hospital, Hank recuperated at home as long as he could, which turned out to be a single restless week. Raring to resume his previous life, he began to climb the walls. Over the objections of his wife and his cardiologist, he returned to his sixty-hour standard workweek. To this day he continues to exhaust himself, pausing only to eat meals rich in saturated fats. He has no intention of taking up exercise or meditation. "I just don't have time," he explains.

My other friend, Thomas, couldn't have responded more differently to his heart attack. "That was as close to sudden death as I'd want to come," he says. "Believe me, it caught my attention, woke me up. I more than slowed down: I retired. If I'd stayed two more years at my job, I'd have collected fuller retirement benefits, but I knew the stress would kill me at my desk before then. My heart attack began to seem like not such a total tragedy; it felt mixed, like being refused passage on the *Titanic.*

"My retirement income isn't huge, but money's not the only currency. Now that I don't work, I'm much richer in time and friendships. I hang out more with my family and friends, do only what I want to do. I relax, I meditate, even loaf and daydream. My wife and I take long walks. My doctor tells me my heart's healing well, so maybe I can begin exercising soon. I'd love to build up to daily running."

Having encountered the same "disease," Hank and Thomas experienced their "illnesses" as oppositely as night and day. Heart attacks being no small business, both men suffered their share of fear, pain, anxiety, and inconvenience, to be sure, but they also attached their own personal interpretations to their respective experiences. It's from these interpretations, not their identical diseases, that Hank acts one way and Thomas another.

When we're sick, we suffer not from our disease, but from our illness—what the disease means to us. That being the case, meaning is as central to healing as the skeleton is to the body. Unlike a body's bones, though, meaning isn't built into sickness: we manufacture it ourselves.

WE GIVE ILLNESS ITS MEANING

Meaning doesn't exist in the physical world. It's entirely a human construct. We make meaning of every event, including sickness. Considering that meanings guide our subsequent behavior, they're real enough, but they're inevitably our own creation.

Too many of us conclude from this notion that we're *entirely* responsible for our own reality, and it's an easy reach from there to claim that we therefore bring on our diseases and suffering. That's not so. It's more accurate to say we co-create our reality: the material world undoubtedly exists, and what we make of it is our choice.

Suppose you and I are taking a walk, and a dog approaches us. Noticing it, we each infuse the event with our personal meanings. I think, Oh, that looks like the nasty cur that bit me when I was four. So I spin around and return sweatily home. And you think, What a neat little doggie, a twin to my long-lost Fluffy. You walk toward the same animal I flee from. Confronted with a single stimulus, we respond differently, based on the meanings we've made of it.

Why we select one particular meaning from a multitude of possibilities is anybody's guess. I prefer to let others argue whether our choice arises from nature or nurture—or from kismet, for that matter—since I suspect the ultimate answer's in permanent fog. All I know is that we derive our meanings in some fashion and store them rather unconsciously, and then they direct our every act. We behave in accordance with our beliefs, and as a matter of fact cannot do otherwise. In fact, to learn anyone's deepest meanings, simply watch her behavior: actions do indeed speak louder than words.

Meaning Creates Suffering

Recall that when you and I encountered that dog, I suffered and you didn't. I felt fear. I fled, though, not because of the dog, but because of what the dog *meant* to me. The meaning you hung on the dog granted you a pleasant emotion, so you stayed and had a fine time.

I recently saw a bumper sticker that advised: PAIN IS INEVITABLE, SUFFERING IS OPTIONAL. This message struck me as a glib but valid shorthand for linking suffering with meaning. Pain hurts enough on its own, yet we often decorate it with intensifying meanings.

As Jack began to drift into sleep one night, thoughts of his friend Ted floated through his mind. Ted had recently been diagnosed with prostate cancer that had spread to his spine. Jack fell asleep but awoke after midnight with a pain in his neck. He thought, Oh, oh. What if it's a tumor? I'll have to see Dr. T. I can't stand Dr. T. If my boss finds out I'm sick, he'll lay me off for sure, and then I'll lose my medical insurance. Where am I going to find the time to write my will? And there's no getting around talking to my ex-wife about the kids' college funds.

As his mind reverberated with such thoughts, Jack's neck pain expanded down into his shoulder and up behind his eyes. With difficulty, he drove himself to an emergency room. The doctor examined him thoroughly, took X-rays, and said, "I think you must've gone to bed with your neck in a funny position."

Jack isn't neurotic. We've all unconsciously aggravated a simple pain by allowing our minds to embellish it with ever-wilder thoughts. Suffering arises from meanings we've applied to a particular situation—what I made of the dog that approached us, what Jack made of his neck pain.

If meaning is the way into suffering, it's also the way out, because healing can begin with a change in meaning. Need I always fear that dog, or can I learn that what happened when I was four won't necessarily recur? Recalling or even imagining just one friendly canine encounter, I won't feel limited to a single response the next time I meet a dog.

The different ways in which Hank and Thomas saw their respective heart attacks aren't engraved on holy stone tablets, either. They had and still have freedom to choose otherwise. Since there are no meanings in this world outside our manufacture, we're always free to drop those that no longer serve us—and may even damage us—and conjure new ones, meanings that are more current, appropriate, and therapeutic.

Of course, I say this naively, as though our meanings were as evident to us as labels on a jar. In real life, they normally abide invisibly and so are seldom accessed. Still, in those instances when we do bring our meanings to awareness, realize them consciously, we can also notice alternatives we didn't select, choices still available to us.

MEANINGS WEAVE A STORY

To learn the nature of your sick friend or relative's suffering—that is, what she makes of her illness—listen to the stories she tells about it.

And tell about it she will, since we're all natural storytellers. Stories may be the hub of humanity's wheel: those of us who have an opposable thumb and walk upright express our meanings continually, much of it in story form.

Indeed, we can't stop. When psychologists experimentally isolate two people in a room with explicit instructions *not* to communicate, the subjects immediately shrug to each other the message "Please excuse me, but we're not supposed to communicate." Then, realizing they've violated instructions with their body language, they show one another their backs, which of course says "No, really, I can't have anything to do with you." Psychologists who watch these futile duets conclude that we're obligate blabbers.

What is this incessant prattle about, anyway? The bulk of it is autobiographical broadcast, some variant of "Here's who I am, what my world is, what I make of my life." Consider how much of your own daily conversation consists of what you've encountered, how you understood and responded to it, the sort of person you are, what the whole adventure means to you. Each of us is a small-time Homer, singing our personal epic within the cultural chorus.

There's something ironic about these epics, though: we don't recognize them until they're out of our mouths. *Only by telling our stories can we understand our meanings.* When I fail to tell them, allow them to stagnate within me, their meanings remain unusably vague. I know this because I heard three fictitious baseball umpires discuss their work.

Umpire One said, "I calls 'em as I sees 'em."

Umpire Two said, "I calls 'em as they *is*."

And Umpire Three said, "Until I calls 'em, they *ain't!*"

Our meanings aren't ours to manipulate unless and until we

express them. The word *meaning* itself comes from Anglo-Saxon *menan*, "to tell." As long as a meaning lurks unseen inside us, we're its unwitting slave: our consequent behavior is unconscious, habitual, automatic. When we bring it to light, though, we can look it over and decide whether we wish to retain it as a director of behavior. This process begins when we realize we're not simply telling *a* story, but telling *our* story and that we *are* the story. Then we can lead it where we like.

I wish we attended to our own stories as relentlessly as we express them. We too easily take them for granted. If we were to listen to them seriously, we'd understand ourselves more deeply since they actually become clearer with repetition. In the same way that a photographic print divulges increasing detail as it develops, stories reveal increasing meaning in their retelling.

LISTENING TO A STORY FOR MEANING

Recall a favorite story from your own past, your *history*, as it were. With each repetition you perfected it, didn't you? You polished highlights, pruned inessentials. Who decided which part of the story was its wheat and which its dispensable chaff? You did. As you retell your story, then, a careful listener will notice from its alterations the relative prominence of its characters and significance of each event. That is, a story is more than a tale: as it changes with repetition it reveals its teller's meanings, attitudes, belief system.

My friend Carol saw her gynecologist because of continual vaginal bleeding. "He found fibroids in my uterus," she told me afterward, "so he did a D&C." (A D&C is dilation and curettage, reaming of the uterine lining.)

A month later, she updated her story. "I've begun bleeding again, off cycle. Feels like there's all this blood in there, churning around."

Another month went by, and she took the story further. "My doctor wanted to do a D&C again. I told him I didn't think peeling my insides every month was a great way to live. This blood just keeps accumulating, wanting to get out. It'd be nice if I could see what's blocking it."

Carol consulted a guided imagery practitioner to help her literally imagine what the metaphorical obstruction might be. She phoned me immediately after the session and exclaimed, "Just as I thought! There was nothing wrong with my uterus. In my mind's eye I saw something around the outside of my cervix, constricting it. And what do you think it was? My wedding ring!"

I didn't know what to say.

She continued, "I knew it! I knew it! I was weeping bloody tears over my stinking marriage!"

Carol stopped seeing her gynecologist and instead saw an attorney and began divorce proceedings. Within two weeks her bleeding stopped.

Note that she began her story from a purely physical perspective, relating the discovery of fibroids and the consequent D&C. As time went on she began to impute a kind of consciousness to her uterine blood: it was "churning"; it "wanted to get out" but something was "blocking" it. Her story came to full fruition when she finally visualized the image that indelibly linked her uterine dysfunction to her marriage.

WE BECOME OUR STORIES

Personal stories mimic the human life cycle. They change most visibly during their infancy. In editing them as we retell them, we bring them to maturity. They gradually gain stability, but at some cost of experiment and passion. By their middle age, our stories are tired, almost drained of their original emotional juice. We know they're finally in their dotage when we tell them in monotone. Our friends thank their stars when we mercifully stop recounting our stiffest, most senile stories.

We put stories to rest not because they're dead and gone but, on the contrary, because we've absorbed them, archived them in our warehouse, which happens to be the body. The more we accept a given story's lessons, the more readily we literally incorporate it, pack it into our flesh. That is, over time our most important stories actually change us physically. As I'll explain in more detail in the next chapter, the body is a vehicle of expression as much as an exhibit of genetic product.

Mark Twain observed, "After thirty, a man is responsible for his face." My friend Spencer was certainly responsible for his. His furrowed brow and serious frown cautioned others not to invade his perpetually profound contemplations. Funny, though: I never heard him say anything even remotely sage. In fact, his sparse comments usually revealed his discomfort with people, his preference for solitude. One day it dawned on me that Spencer's countenance, rather than reflecting deep thought, served to convey to others the impression of preoccupation precisely so they'd leave him alone.

The body is more than our instrument of behavior. It's also the means by which we perceive the world. We're permeated by tiny organs that detect touch, smell, position, image, taste, pressure, temperature, moisture, sound, pain, and, I'm sure, other modalities we haven't identified yet. Our stories, as they subtly alter our physical configuration, must influence as well the operation of our sense organs, and so modify our perceptions, filter our experiences.

That is, we sense the world and then respond to it as our preconceptions dictate. With every passing year, we inhabit a reality increasingly of our own devise. Ultimately, the phrase *I'll believe it when I see it* becomes truer when reversed. The notion, then, that saints walk in beauty is less a pretty metaphor than a concrete truth: each of our worlds is very much what it seems to us.

THE ILLNESS STORY AS A PATH TO HEALING

If our stories reveal something of the reality we each occupy, then the stories we tell about our illnesses can reveal the precise nature of our suffering and, within that, the key to its alleviation.

To listen with an ear toward healing demands that we respect the special characteristics of illness stories.

- First, they seem to follow a general pattern of devastation, reflection, and response. (It's helpful to be aware of this pattern, but we'll need to let it go in order to hear the *uniqueness* in our loved one's story.)

- Second, illness stories, consisting as they do of both fact and imagination, constitute a wider truth than fact alone. We're rational beings only in part, so complete understanding must honor our irrational aspect as well.

- Third, like dreams, these stories can beg interpretation, a challenge that demands skillful handling. For what relief it may offer you, know now that you don't have to interpret anything.

- Fourth, illness stories are spun around an emotional core. It's important to identify this core, since it holds energy useful for therapeutic change.

- And finally, the style of telling most likely to lead to healing is precisely the style the teller chooses.

ILLNESS STORIES USUALLY EXHIBIT DEVASTATION, REFLECTION, AND RESPONSE

Ada, who was seventy years old, lived in a board-and-care home. During a routine physical exam, her doctor diagnosed an isolated breast tumor. Two days later she had a mastectomy. She recovered rapidly, but when she returned to the home, she was depressed.

Edith, Ada's best friend, who lived across the hall, knocked on her door. "Ada, it's me."

"Can't talk now," was the response, followed by muffled crying.

Edith left Ada alone then. Several days later, over tea, she asked her, "So how's your healing going?"

"Terrible. What do I have to offer anyone?" Ada answered. "I'm old. Dried up. Sick, too."

"Gee, I felt like that when I had my mastectomy."

Ada was surprised. "I didn't know you'd had a mastectomy."

"Oh, yes." Edith smiled, then changed the subject.

They spoke together daily, Ada about the feelings her operation raised, and Edith about her similar history.

After a week, Ada said, "You know, I'm kind of angry at myself. You handled your mastectomy better than I'm handling mine."

"But, Ada, I had mine long ago. Yours was only last month. I was in terrible shape right after mine."

"Still, Edith, it seems you know there's more to you than breasts. Why should it be that losing a breast makes so much difference to me now?"

"Well, I'm not surprised you feel that way, but you tell me. Why should it?"

Ada pondered. "I guess if I live much longer I could lose other organs, too. I better consider exactly who I am besides . . ." she tapped her chest ". . . this stuff."

Ada and Edith continued to meet almost daily. Meanwhile, Ada privately went through her photo collection at home to remind herself of what her life had been. She reestablished contact with both her children, who'd been repulsed by her depression.

A few weeks later she announced to Edith, "All these conversations we've had make me think now that maybe I can experiment a little. So I want to let you know something. I'm thinking about having a breast reconstruction."

Ada paused, looked down, blushed, and continued, "I've met a very nice gentleman, a little younger than me, as a matter of fact. But that isn't why I'm having my reconstruction. He says he doesn't care a bit. It's me who wants it. Can't a seventy-year-old feel glamorous?"

Ada's story began as a wordless, depressed, *devastated* cry. Passing through that feeling, she began to tell a story of *reflection*, what her disease meant to her, and Edith encouraged her to do so by means of her skillful conversation. Gradually Ada recognized the place her disease and its treatment occupied in her life, what it caused her to believe about herself, and what sort of options she might consider.

Finally she *responded*, speaking of blossoming into a new life. Now she says, "I used to fear my cancer all the time. I still think about it some, but it's less negative, more like wondering. Was my depression actually telling me to abandon my old life and enter this new one? I even wonder whether I would have made any of the changes I've made if it hadn't been for cancer."

Ada well exemplified the general, three-part pattern. *The initial form most illness stories take is flat-out devastation.* My life is gone, it's all over, there's nothing to look forward to. People usually tell their story this way for a week or two, provided they're not so shattered they can't speak at all.

The second form is reflection. The explosion's shock waves are spent. The worst has happened. My life as I knew it is gone. Funny, though: I'm still here. Who have I become? What's my current reality? How shall I proceed?

The final form is response. I realize it's an all-new game. My days were always numbered, but now that I know that for a certainty, I'm going to milk them for all they're worth. I can even entertain the possibility of a life better than what I had before I got sick.

To appreciate how an illness story evolves, think of a misfortune from your past. It needn't be a sickness. How did you go through your divorce, your accident, the loss of a job? At any given time, the story you told had a flavor of devastation, reflection, or response, so that a careful listener could track your progress from suffering through healing.

Now that I've described that basic story pattern, I'll ask you to respect its many exceptions. Story styles run the gamut from disorganized graffiti to mythic sagas that Joseph Campbell could have dictated. I resist offering firm categorization because, frankly, I dread this book falling into the wrong hands: there are those who, preferring theory to reality, will push a story through some ideologic filter and thereby mangle it. So regard the pattern I outlined only as a generalization. People can and do depart from it.

Andre, a young law student, developed Hodgkin's disease. He said, "I learned I had it in December, got treated on weekends, and didn't miss a day of school. Now it's May, and cancer's just another item on my plate, not much worse than my contracts exam."

Following his finals in June, though, he crashed. He spiraled into a depression so deep that there was no question of his returning to school for the fall term. *Devastated* a half-year after his diagnosis, he chose to go on an antidepressant. In November, when he was finally off the drug, Andre *reflected,* "It took me all this time to realize how big cancer is. But back then? I think I was out of my mind *not* to have been blown away. When my counselor recently told me, 'Buried feelings are always buried alive,' I sure knew what she meant. You can't avoid feelings, only delay them. You eventually have to repay loans . . . and with interest, too.

"During most of my life I repressed certain feelings so I could go on living a style I thought suited me. Now I see that style as actually *preventing* the life I really need to lead."

Andre's *response* was to obtain an indefinite leave of absence from his studies. The rest of that school year he sat quietly at home, thought about his life, and attended a cancer support group. Now, two years later, he's in remission and has a job in a bookstore. He advises cancer novices, "I'm still not entirely certain where I'm going. Maybe I'll go back to law school, but I suspect I need a more relaxed path. Everyone's got to find their own way. In my life, I've learned that begins by honoring whatever I feel."

ILLNESS STORIES ARE TRUE

All illness stories are true, regardless of their factuality.

My friend Ralph's fiancée, Anita, informed him she was leaving him. Although their breakup had simmered for months, this wasn't at all what Ralph wanted to hear. An hour after she told him her decision, a pain tore through his chest. He wondered aloud if he was having a heart attack. Alarmed, Anita demanded that he see a doctor and drove him to a nearby emergency room.

"I have this pain," he told the doctor. "I'm worried it's my heart."

After examining and thoroughly testing Ralph, the doctor said, "Your heart's perfectly normal. There's nothing wrong with you."

But there was, and Ralph himself had diagnosed it accurately. The problem wasn't in his heart-as-circulatory-pump but in his heart-as-seat-of-emotions. Sometimes we suffer physical injury to the heart muscle, sometimes the arrows of heartache.

Whether an illness story represents, or even claims to represent, hard fact is irrelevant. Writing instructors who teach fiction standardly define their genre as a lie by which we know the truth. William Blake put it nicely: "Ev'rything that is capable of being believ'd is an image of truth." The truth, the Whole Truth—the truth we live by—merges verifiable fact with fantasies from our inner, twilight world. By means of her story, the sick person is trying her best to relate exactly who she is, what her illness means to her, and, coded within that, what might be her route toward healing. To be sure, some stories are more powerful—more spectacular, compelling, inspirational—than others, but all, in their way, are true.

ILLNESS STORIES ARE INTERPRETABLE, but ONLY by THEIR TELLER

We awake in the morning, roll over in bed, and say to our partner, "I had this dream. Tell me what you think it means." Generally aware that we're too immersed in our own mind-play to evaluate it clearly, we ask for help.

Like dreams, illness stories beg explication by others, so don't be surprised if your friend or relative asks you to interpret hers. It's a seductive request: you, too, want to know what her story is "really" about, and you'll be credited as insightful if you're the one who unravels it. But please remember that when you shift your focus from pure listening to interpretation, you've left her, you've lost the healing connection, and are swimming around in your own mind instead.

In addition, you can't know whether your interpretation is accurate. But even if it were absolutely, certifiably guaranteed accurate, it's still your interpretation, whereas the only interpretation she can act upon effectively is her own.

My friend Kirsten, a professional jazz singer, had an aneurysm, a bulging, weak-walled artery, in her liver. Her doctor recommended immediate surgery.

"Oh, I don't think I'm ready for surgery," Kirsten replied.

"What's the problem?"

"Well, actually, I'm not sure. I have to give it a little thought."

She drove directly to the home of her pianist, Brian, and she and Brian discussed her dilemma.

"I know I need surgery," she said, "but I want to do it when I'm ready, and there's something about it that puts me off."

Brian thought awhile and asked, "What do you think the surgery will be like?"

"Well, from what the surgeon told me, I guess the anesthetist will start an IV, give me some kind of tranquilizer, and put a mask over my nose and mouth. And then I'll be out. The surgeon will begin operating. I pretty much won't be there because I'll be unconscious."

Brian said, "Funny, that sure isn't how you and I work together. Every time we've rehearsed, you've micromanaged every note."

"Well, that's just how I am. I have to be in control."

Late that night she awoke suddenly from a deep sleep, unable to breathe. "It was like I couldn't remember how," she told Brian the next day. "Scariest feeling I've ever had. I couldn't make my lungs work."

"Then what happened?"

"I must've been dreaming about control, having and not having it, and I guess my body pushed that all the way. I was totally out of control, actually beginning to black out. Thank God it occurred to me that when I'd been asleep, my breath happened on its own. So as hard as it was, I lay back and relaxed, just let my body take over, and right away, a breath came."

"Wow!" Brian said, and paused. "Why do you suppose that happened to you?"

"Well, I guess I had to feel how much I need to control things, and maybe this surgery's an opportunity for me to make a change. I already know I'm great at control; now I'm asking myself whether I can balance that by *letting* things happen, too."

When Kirsten met with her anesthetist, she asked to insert her own preferences into procedures wherever possible. He agreed to an acupuncture treatment before anesthesia induction and to play Bach to her through headphones during the operation. Negotiating other details with her surgeon, she gradually felt adequate balance between surrender and control, had the operation, and recovered uneventfully.

As we understandably seek interpretation, we may confuse personal meaning with cause. Upon getting sick, we can ask ourselves, "Does this disease mean I was exposed to toxins?" or "Does it mean I have defective genes?" Beware of this tendency, since it's likely to lead more toward guilt than to healing. We tend naturally to search for cause. Inhabiting a science-oriented society, we have little tolerance for uncertainty and so demand to know *why* things happened, why we got sick.

With rare exceptions, though, we'll never know the cause of any given instance of sickness. Statistics, which can suggest cause within large groups, are by definition inapplicable to individuals. Though I'm as convinced as anyone that smoking statistically "causes" lung cancer, I nevertheless know people with lung cancer who've never smoked and know as well that most heavy smokers don't have lung cancer.

Often, people seek the cause of their sickness to reassure themselves that *they* weren't the cause. I've found self-blame to be astonishingly high on people's list of possible causes for their sicknesses.

My friend Julianne reflects, "When I learned my lupus had pretty well fried my kidneys, I was destroyed for weeks. No one could cheer me up. I couldn't even lift my spirits enough to play with my young son.

"It was touch and go, but the doctors finally decided I didn't need kidney dialysis. They put me on heavy steroids for a couple of months. I gained weight. My face puffed out like a full moon. I was a mess.

"When they cut back on the drugs, things got more stable. I began to write my thoughts in a journal, several pages a day. I jabbered away. I didn't know what was important and what wasn't, so I wrote everything that came into my mind. After a month, I went back and read it all. I saw a few themes: my fear, my love of my son, and something peculiar, that business about my kidneys.

"I'd written in a few places that lupus had burned or cooked my kidneys, and about a 'fire in my guts,' and then I came across a passage about wanting to push my ex-husband, Peter, into an oven. Don't worry, I'm not really going to. All those images of fiery anger made me wonder: was I 'pissed off' in my kidneys or in my life?

"I read my journal to my friend Clare, who has lupus, too. She said, 'Now, I don't think you ought to get into who caused what. You'll make yourself believe you attacked your own kidneys, and then you'll feel guilty.'

"She had a point. I didn't need more guilt in my life, but the question of whether I brought this on began to fascinate me. I read a lot about health, so I know people can nudge some diseases along with their behavior. Ulcers can be caused by stress, and heart disease can come from a bad diet and no exercise. If I was furious at Peter and kept it in my body instead of acting it out, wasn't it me, then, who injured my kidneys? Should I feel guilty? Am I a jerk?"

Julianne bought a popular book that implied a causative relationship between attitudes and a variety of disorders. Along with linking arthritis to stubbornness and lung disease to needing to get something off one's chest, the author confirmed that kidney disease was related to unexpressed anger.

"That made me feel supremely guilty," Julianne recalled. "Guilt became all I thought about. When it finally began to drive me nuts, I told Clare I needed to talk about it, so we both got into it. As a matter of fact, she thought she'd done some things that made her lupus worse, too.

"But over several conversations, we realized everybody eats and exercises and makes decisions and manages stress in their way, and every decision has its consequences. In the long run, how we live helps determine how we get sick and die, and everybody, no matter how they live, comes to the end of their road. There's no reason to feel guilty about being human.

"So did I cause my lupus flare? God only knows. Maybe I added to it, maybe not. But one thing Clare and I are both certain of is that we did the best we could do at the time. If I wasn't as openly angry with Peter as I should've been, it was because I didn't know better then, and I do now. However people believe they might have contributed to their sickness, they did their momentary best. They deserve to forgive themselves for how they were, and act now with whatever wisdom they've learned since."

Julianne handled the issue as well as anyone can. A friend of mine who happens to be a world-class healer maintains a list of saints from various spiritual paths who've had cancer. These saints did nothing "wrong" except be mortal, and so be subject, like the rest of us, to sickness and eventually to death.

People who insist on determining the cause of their sickness encounter a pair of pitfalls. First, if they conclude that they themselves created their sickness, they can plummet into a mire of guilt, a course that does no one much good. Second, their energy, which could drive healing action in the present, goes instead toward obsessively—and futilely—untangling their past.

I suggest to sick people that they shift their understanding of responsibility from shades of blame to "response-ability," the ability to respond. As civil rights advocate Jesse Jackson likes to point out, when you're lying in the street after being bumped by a truck, you'll find it less useful to wonder about the make of the truck than to get yourself up off the street.

ILLNESS STORIES CONTAIN POWERFUL EMOTIONS

Stories in general transmit feelings. We remember a story for its meaning—its "moral," we say—and more deeply, for the feelings it ignites in us. A well-told story emotionally connects teller and listener, and listeners with one another. We treasure tales that leave us happy and inspired, to be sure, but no more than those that leave us wistful, frightened, sad, self-righteous, or nostalgic. Whether we're telling about Julianne's anger, Dorothy in the Land of Oz, or the churlish clerk at the Shop-n-Swipe, we're "sharing feelings," as we Californians say, and loving it. If stories were a drug, we'd be junkies.

Our important issues are by definition those we feel emotional about. Over decades, though, we tend to decorate the original emotion with such a thick verbal filigree—reasons, associations, rationalizations—that we lose track of what was first there. If we talk about these issues to someone who listens well, we can eventually recover (more accurately, *un*cover) the pure emotion. At that point, when we're actively emoting instead of caught in our thinking mind, we'll begin to respond to the situation as it originally affected us. Our healing journey aims ultimately at the center of our suffering, or what I called in a previous chapter Job's whirlwind. Our most effective response to our illness will be the one that originates emotionally.

Philip Roth's *Portnoy's Complaint* offers an excellent example of this process. The book is entirely the protagonist's tragicomic lament to his psychiatrist. Portnoy goes on for hundreds of pages, without a word from his listener, until, having finally said all he can possibly say, he's reduced to screams and moans, raw emotion. Only then does the Vienna-born psychiatrist speak, and his is the last line in the book: "Now we may perhaps to begin."

Think of your sick friend or relative's illness story as a protective, civilizing insulation around her emotion. As your relationship with her, and consequently her trust, deepens, she'll gingerly peel away the story until only the emotion remains. That emotion is the passion that will drive her healing behavior.

Monique, who had stomach cancer, has now been in remission for a year. She sees her oncologist every month for routine monitoring. After a recent visit, she told her friend Irene, "I don't know why he keeps me in that waiting room so long, at least an hour and a half every time. If he knows it's going to be that long, why doesn't he schedule me ninety minutes later?"

"How's that make you feel, Monique?" Irene asked.

"Well, hmmm. It makes me feel victimized, like I'm weak, too sick to fight back."

"Are you too sick to fight back?"

"No, damn it, I'm not." Monique stood up.

"Wow! You sound . . ."

"Royally furious!" She punched her palm.

A few weeks later, Monique told Irene, "When I saw my doctor last week, I purposely showed up ninety minutes late. The receptionist looked at me like she expected some excuse, but I said, 'I'm deliberately late today, the same amount of time the doctor always has me wait. I'm not going to put up with that anymore. My time's valuable to me. Making me wait so long is disrespectful.' I still can't believe I actually said that. Anyway, she disappeared for a minute, then came back to the window and showed me into an examining room. The doctor came right in and fell all over himself apologizing. He said he hadn't realized how long I'd waited and promised from then on to give me a realistic appointment time."

ILLNESS STORIES MUST BE TOLD AS THEIR TELLERS WISH

Of the many seriously sick people with whom I've worked, the ones who do best, all else being equal, are those who enter their chosen treatment wholeheartedly. In *Love, Medicine and Miracles* and his ensuing books, Dr. Bernie Siegel emphasizes that the people who fight their cancers most effectively are those who insist on gathering information independently, making up their own minds, and plotting their own course, sometimes a course that looks unorthodox to others. Depending on which direction they're seen from, they're either the "worst" patients or, as Siegel prefers to call them, "exceptional." Strongly agreeing with

Siegel, I've found exceptionality enhanced when people are encouraged to tell their stories their way. If they don't relate the beginning, middle, or end we'd prefer, that's our problem, not theirs.

Sixty-year-old Jack said, "I got colon cancer five years ago. When they removed it, they found it'd spread to some lymph nodes. The doctors gave me chemo but it made me so sick, they backed off and said maybe they'd treat it more aggressively later.

"It felt like my life was gone. I got depressed, just sat around. One day my wife happened to point out that however long I'd be alive, I was running out the clock moping. That got to me, so maybe when a friend told me about meditation, I was ready. I went to some classes, discovered it did something for me. I began to practice every day. I heard maybe it was a way to stimulate my immune system. I don't know if meditation does that, but it did bring me peace. It did something else, too. I saw the world a little differently afterward. Fresher, maybe. Or maybe it was me who was fresher.

"A year after my first diagnosis, they discovered I had prostate cancer, too. This time I had some tools, though. I researched prostate cancer, got copies of my medical records, surfed the Internet, got a bunch of opinions. One doctor wanted to operate, another recommended hormones and radiation. I weighed it all and decided on the course they call watchful waiting, which means I was simply going to monitor the situation.

"My decision gave a couple of the doctors and a lot of my friends and relatives the willies. They couldn't understand why somebody with two cancers would opt for no medical treatment. They phoned me, begged me, bugged me, probably even lost sleep over it.

"But I'm not doing nothing, only nothing medical. Fact is, I do plenty. Every morning I wake up at four, make myself a cup of essiac tea, meditate, pray, and do my ta'i chi. Then it's off to work. I hesitated telling the guys on the job site about my routine, afraid they'd make fun of me. Actually, though, they're amazed how well it works for me. My wife sees that, too, and congratulates me every day. I must say my cancers—or maybe it's all these practices I do now—changed my life for the better."

To invite people to tell their story their way—to honor their style, content, direction, asides, decisions, and conclusions—is to accelerate their healing. That's not easy to do, especially when we think we've heard this tale before and know its ending, or know we'd do differently. When we feel this way, it's usually because we've forgotten how much of our delight with stories depends on surprise. Expectations blunt stories, pare them toward the generic, so we must keep in mind that each is unique, and every telling fresh.

If you need scientific confirmation of that principle, consider what happened when researchers wired a Zen master to an electroencephalograph, a machine that records brain waves. They asked the master to meditate, then watched as his brain waves slowed in frequency, an objective sign of relaxation. Suddenly and without warning, a screaming stranger burst into the room. The researchers had intentionally planned this surprise to see what would happen to the master's brain waves. The waves quickened immediately, indicating that the intrusion had indeed disturbed him. No big news here. The researchers escorted the stranger out. They apologized to the master and asked him to regain serenity, and soon his brain waves evinced relaxation. Then the stranger burst in screaming once again, and here's where things got interesting. One would expect the master to "learn"—that is, display less brain wave disturbance—with each interruption. But he didn't: no matter how many times the screamer entered, the master's degree of neurologic upheaval remained consistent. Was he ineducable? No, he explained: every event is unique.

To favor a particular ending for a story is to assume that our notion of healing, wonderfully valid though it looks to us, will work for someone else. Recall from the beginning of this chapter how Hank and Thomas responded to their heart attacks. Which response would you have chosen, Hank's resignation or Thomas's hope? Thomas's impresses me as the healthier, and I'll bet you agree.

If you're to help either man heal, though, it's important to acknowledge your preference, whatever it is, and then relinquish it promptly, for it will limit you: only Hank and Thomas themselves can determine whether they're on their "right" route. Since Hank's heart attack obviously wasn't his wake-up call, maybe he needs to return to his accustomed overwork to attract the event that *will* capture his attention. That catalyst might be anything from a saronged siren who bears him off to Tahiti, to a friend's offhand comment about key lime pie. Sadly, his sudden death may arrive first. As fervently as we might wish Hank to amend his "type A," hard-driving personality, we must be prepared for the possibility that he'll ignore all omens, never even approach the emotional charge that might initiate his healing. For that matter, how sure are we that Thomas made the "right" choice? Do we know he won't set out on his first fitness run and get flattened by an errant bulldozer? Given that we can't know Hank's or Thomas's existential destinations, how certain can we be of the route they should take?

Sick people's responses may not always seem advisable, sensible, or even sane to us. But we must keep in mind that behind closed doors we behave idiosyncratically. Perhaps you'll recall the massive study *Human Sexual Response*, authored in 1966 by William Masters and Virginia Johnson. I've always treasured one of their conclusions:

> There are so many variables of sexual response that no possibility exists for establishing norms of sexual performance . . . [1]

The authors were as surprised as their readers to learn that in matters of sex, everyone does pretty much whatever he or she likes.

We're similarly willful when sick: when we realize that all the cards are finally on the table, we do precisely what we like. Although I'm a trained scientist, I'm no more immune to that phenomenon than anyone else. Several years ago I addressed my own serious disorder in ways that, though apparently effective, struck many of my medical colleagues as demented. I can't predict my response to my next episode, except to promise that it will depend on the exigencies of the moment. Fascinatingly strange beings that we are, we must act as we see fit at the time. I told you about Hank and Thomas not to endorse or condemn their choices, then, but to ask how much flexibility *you* can develop in allowing them to tell their stories in their own way.

An inherent part of a story's style is the pace with which it's told. Having evolved over substantial time, it's of intricate construction, so must be unfolded delicately. There's no schedule for the elaboration of a story, any more than there's a proper date to end grief. One illness explorer will sniff out revelations from the start while another stammers for months.

Besides, I know from personal experience that our first several sentences or even paragraphs can amount to little more than throat-clearing. Our opening words are often dully habitual, and only when we press beyond them do we arrive at something more vital, perhaps something we've never said before. It's a longer distance to the mouth from the heart than from the head, so heartfelt speech takes a little longer. A genuine healing room, then, contains these inhabitants: the patient and the *patient*.

TO HEAL

1. Encourage your sick friend or relative to tell you the story of her illness, from the beginning. "What's it been like for you?" "What's been the most important part of your sickness?" "What have you made of all this?"

2. Recognize her devastation. She may initially be in such turmoil that she's unable to do more than be emotional. You can help here by assuring her that her intense feelings are a normal response.

3. Note emotions in her story. As she speaks, watch for the parts of her story that seem sad, angry, or emotional in some other way. After she finishes, ask her to elaborate those areas. "I'd like to hear more about when you told your mother you had a life-threatening disease . . ." "Can you say what you felt when your doctor told you that you had diabetes?"

(continued)

"How did you feel when your children said they didn't want to hear about your cancer?"

4. Resist the temptation to interpret her story. Avoid interpretation even if she requests it of you. The only useful meanings in her story are *hers.* To help her clarify them, ask her questions like "What did you make of that tightness in your chest?" or "What did your dream about removing your bandage mean to you?"

5. Focus on her current emotions. She may persist in looking to the past to determine what caused her sickness—or what she did "wrong"—rather than explore what it means to her now. Without interrupting, ask her gently about her current feelings. "How does the guilt you told me about affect you right now?" "How do you feel about not knowing the cause of your disease [or prospects for your future]?"

6. Let her tell her story her way. Recognize and abandon any preferences you have for how her story should progress. Don't guess at what she'll say, and never finish her sentences. Let her story surprise you.

FIVE

Using Your Ears, Eyes, and Heart

> *People tell their illness stories with*
> *their entire being.*

To treat a man as something to which surgery, drugs, and hoodoo applied was an indifferent matter; to treat him as material for a work of art made him somehow come alive to me.
—William Carlos Williams, *Autobiography*

A man's face, as a rule, says more and more interesting things than his mouth.
—Arthur Schopenhauer

There's More to Expression than Speech
One of my psychiatry professors regularly conducted a magic show for the medical students.

Every Wednesday, four new students attended his interview of a patient he'd never before met. Psychiatrists are notorious for asking questions that can seem silly. "Who's the president of the United States?" they'll ask, and "What does *A rolling stone gathers no moss* mean?" He did none of that. For ten minutes, he and the patient simply chatted about the lunch of creamed chipped beef and the bingo game in the dayroom. Then the professor thanked the patient, showed him back to the ward, and began to tell us the man's entire biography.

"Mr. LaSalle was born near New Orleans. Not in, but near; he's got the accent but no urban patina. He was an only child, by the way: he resents not being the center of attention now, so I imagine he got pretty much what he wanted as a kid. Judging from his slight edge of impatience, I'd say he dropped out of high school before graduating. He joined the Navy. No big deal; you saw the tattoo. Eventually he married a woman I'd guess is Asian, probably Japanese or Okinawan, considering the time. Did you see his almost imperceptible bow when he entered the room? Anyway, he's divorced now. You noticed the pale band of skin around his left fourth finger . . ."

And on he went for half an hour. When at last he finished, he summoned the ward psychiatrist, who read from Mr. LaSalle's chart. The two histories could have been carbon copies.

We'd known to expect this tour de force, so legendary was the professor's perceptivity. During the interview, while he sat comfortably, we perched at the edge of our chairs fairly vibrating with vigilance. Sure, we heard the man's accent and saw his tattoo, but in our strained attentiveness we missed much else and in any event were too choked to put it all together.

Afterward, we hounded him for his secret. He told us what he told all the others: "Listen to the music, not the words."

For years, that advice abided in me as one of those ideas-that-ring-true-but-I-don't-quite-get. Only when I began to consider it literally did it make sense. Human expression so exuberantly transcends words that we must conceive it in wider terms. Some authors liken it to music, even to the point of suggesting that we virtually *are* music. In his fascinating book *Meaning and Medicine*, Dr. Larry Dossey proposes

> a radically different image of the body: that it is not a machine, as we have been told, but music, down to the actual atoms and molecules that comprise it. A new picture emerges: the body as an enchanted instrument on which mind and meaning play. The metaphor of the musical body . . . is not only consistent with certain spiritual insights that have developed through the ages, but also has been put forward by serious scientists.

Let's try that metaphor. Think of your sick friend or relative's illness story as an operetta, a composition blending text with tune. In this view the lyrics are his verbal language. His music includes his emotional tone, location, posture, gestures, movements, stillnesses, dress, ornament, and even aroma—that is, everything he expresses nonverbally. Each word and musical note and every rest between them is significant.

First, Sense the Person's Mood

A sick friend or relative's operetta begins with a wordless overture, his emotional tone. Before he utters a sound, he sets his stage with his dominant current mood. His mood can be so subtle I won't notice it unless I approach him mindfully. (Indeed, I'll appreciate every aspect of his expression most acutely when I'm quietly mindful.) Besides, my initial silence signifies respect for his extraordinary state, sickness. My first glimpse—my initial impression of him and his *ambiance*—ought to convey some sense of his mood.

In his book *Vital Signs,* Dr. Fitzhugh Mullan touchingly describes the healing that can come from noting a sick person's emotional tone. While a U.S. Public Health Service physician, Mullan developed a galloping cancer that required extensive treatment at the National Naval Medical Center. Weeks later, after having suffered both his disease and almost every misfortune that can befall one in a hospital, he sank into a depression. Alarmed at Mullan's state, his doctor requested a psychiatric consultation.

Mullan writes that at that point he felt absolutely hopeless, and certainly pessimistic about what a Navy psychiatrist might offer.

The psychiatrist entered Mullan's room. He took a long look at him. Then, without a word, he sat on Mullan's bed and held him. Mullan reports that moment to have been the beginning of his recovery, and today he's a prominent cancer patient advocate.

Sometimes the simple act of compassionately witnessing someone's suffering is the only healing he needs. My psychiatry professor would have suggested that the more thoroughly we listen to the sick person's "music," the less we need to rely on words at all.

My friend Nancy told me, "I visited my sister Lydia, who'd just been diagnosed with lung cancer. She and I have always been close, and we live only a couple of miles apart. I figured maybe I could lift her spirits.

"Her bedroom door was open, so I peeked in. Lydia was folded up in a corner of her bed, awake, and totally still. For some reason, I got the feeling she was frightened, even afraid to move. She smiled at me, but painfully, like it took all her energy.

"We'd been raised not to show any emotion. Whenever I got

angry as a child, my parents said, 'Don't be angry.' Or if Lydia said, 'I'm sad,' they'd tell her there was nothing to be sad about. I realized in my twenties this wasn't healthy, so I saw a counselor for a year, and now I'm actually pretty comfortable with my emotions.

"As I stood in Lydia's bedroom doorway, I wondered for a second what I ought to say. I heard my mother's voice in my head, smoothing things over for my sister. It said, 'Oh, Lydia, don't be scared. Everything's going to be all right.' Luckily, that drifted right away. Besides, I realized, anybody as frightened as Lydia looked couldn't hear anything anyway.

"So I sat on the bed with her. She leaned toward me, put her head in my lap, and started to cry. I even heard myself think, *Don't cry, Lydia,* but I didn't say that. Lydia needed to be scared then, and to cry. I held her and stroked her hair for ten minutes, and slowly, her rigidity seemed to leave her body along with her tears. Finally she sat up, and then we talked plenty."

Note the Sick Person's Appearance

Having entered your friend or relative's room and sensed his mood, notice where he is in the room and what he's doing. If he's in bed, is he lying comfortably or does he look exhausted? Is he twisting in pain or curled into a fetal position? Is he working at a desk? Looking contemplatively out the window? Watching television? Is he holding forth, in the role of host, or is he withdrawn?

When he stands, does he attain his full height, or is he bent with care, pain, or depression? How quickly and how confidently does he move? Are his gestures expansive, restricted, or even absent?

How is he dressed? Is he wearing a hospital-issue gown? If he's in his own clothing, is it because he insisted on his individuality?

Are his clothes clean? He may be content to wear soiled or decrepit garments if he's depressed. What might flashy clothes say about him? Does his haircut proclaim him to be vain, dramatic, faddish, businesslike? Does he wear jewelry, tattoos, or other features intended to beautify, declare, or outrage?

What smells do you notice? In some cultures, people sniff one another unabashedly for elements that sight, hearing, and touch can't detect. Although we're not as well practiced, most of us can smell whether a total stranger is, say, an auto mechanic, a baker, or a cigarette smoker. And I know a few people who claim, reliably, I think, that they can smell fear, anger, and seductiveness.

Emotional tone, appearance, style, and even smell, then, make up some of your sick friend or relative's music. Now let's consider his body itself.

Note His Body Language

Often more accurate than words, our body holds forth by means of its position and movements, to be sure, but also with its very shape.

Long ago, my two-year-old daughter asked a question as provocative as it was childish. During a dinner party, she turned to a guest and asked, "Why do you look like that?" Though the poor man was actually quite presentable, he made a courteous exit, checked his teeth for spinach, and returned, no less unnerved.

Why *do* we look the way we do? Certainly, some body-shaping forces, such as genes, are outside our control. But we made our own lifelong contributions, too, by means of habitual behaviors that gradually altered our appearance. If actions speak louder than words, then repetitive actions—habits—express even deeper beliefs. One useful way to see the body, then, is as a complete autobiographical portfolio. Laid over my core of genetically dictated features are certain ways I've chosen to live my life, and it's all to be seen for the looking.

Habit changes our physical form. Perform any act repetitively and the involved muscles grow. Which of your arms is larger, the one that raises the bowling ball and swings the tennis racquet, or the other one? Who has larger leg muscles, a runner or a sedentary office worker? Thus the biologist's dictum, "Form follows function."

The reverse is as true: use it or lose it. Remember when your doctor removed the cast from your healing broken leg? The limb looked ghastly, didn't it? Having been out of commission for weeks, your muscles had shrunk. But as you began to use the leg again, it regained its healthy size.

Physicians have long recognized repetitive behavior's influence on physique with their curious Latin word for body shape, *habitus.* Habits aren't random. We enact them purposefully, however unconsciously, and the body gradually transforms in response to those habits.

My friend Raymond was unhappy. One evening, chatting over a beer with his co-worker Mitch, he said, "I don't know what it is. I can't put my finger on it. I'm just plain miserable." He paused. "Well, actually, I suspect it has something to do with my size." Raymond weighed more than three hundred pounds.

"What's your weight got to do with your misery?" Mitch asked.

"I don't understand what you're asking."

"Well, let me ask you this way: what does your body feel like to you?"

"What do you mean? Do I like myself? Do I feel unhealthy?"

"No, not your conclusions, something simpler: how does your body feel to you? What's it like to live in there? Can you compare it to something, paint me a picture?"

Raymond thought. "Well, it feels heavy. No surprise, I guess. But it feels heavy like an anchor."

"An anchor?"

"Yeah, like it keeps me grounded. If it didn't press me down, I'd drift away."

"And then?"

"I'd lift off into the ozone. I'm a dreamer, Mitch. You've seen me at work. I make all kinds of crazy plans without considering reality. I'd be lost without practical people like you around me. My brothers always called me an airhead, and I think they were right."

Mitch gave this some thought. "Yeah, I can understand how it'd feel that way to you, then."

Raymond asked, "Well, isn't it so?"

"Who knows what's so? Frankly, though, that isn't the way I see you."

"So tell me. How do you see me?"

"As creative and, as a matter of fact, just as practical. Maybe who your brothers saw when you were younger and who you are now aren't the same person."

They spoke further, but in this short conversation Raymond began to understand for the first time what his body shape meant to him. Over the next few months, he continued to speak about it to Mitch and other close friends. Without adopting any particular diet, he lost eighty pounds in a year and for the first time in a decade began to date.

He recently told me, "When I was a kid, I really was a hopeless dreamer, but I don't think that's the whole story now. I still dream, but it just might be that I'm as grounded as anybody else. Maybe I don't need to clutch the Earth as much as I used to."

Raymond's body is no more expressive than yours or mine. We all make physical comments. Imagine that you work at a job you despise, under a supervisor invented by Dickens in a dark mood. Whenever you hear him slither behind you, you raise your shoulders in the primitive reflex that protects your vulnerable throat from predators. As you unconsciously lift your shoulders twenty times daily, you begin to develop impressive definition in your trapezius muscles. Form follows function: with time, your shoulders at rest are steadily higher. Do this exercise until, say, retirement age, and you'll find your shoulders lifted permanently. At that point you'll attend a dinner party where a two-year-old asks you, "Why do you look like that?" and you'll shrug, "Genes, I guess." Nope. Your habit has become your shape.

Our very bodies, then, help express the meanings with which we live. Going through life stoop-shouldered may announce that you feel the weight of the world. A downturned mouth may say silently that you've found much of life distasteful. If the opposite sex glances pleasingly whenever you hold your body in a particular configuration, you'll likely hold it that way more often, and eventually you'll forget how to hold it any other way. Our most habitual habits, so to speak, can progressively take us over, mold our shapes to better serve *them*.

As with Raymond, though, the meaning that drives a habitus can outlive its usefulness. At that point, it becomes a waste of energy at best, and at worst a tilt toward physical disorder.

Paul, a college professor, developed neck pain resulting from spinal arthritis. One afternoon, the department secretary, Moira, found Paul at his desk, wincing as he massaged his neck.

"Your arthritis?"

"Aaaaaagh."

do you feel now, Paul?"

do you mean? It just hurts."

me what it feels like."

"Ah, it feels . . . well, contracted, like it's being pulled into my chest."

"It's being pulled in?"

"Like *I'm* pulling it in. I feel like I'm a damn turtle going into my shell, if you want to know."

"Why into your shell?" Moira asked. "What's outside?"

"Thanks, Moira, but frankly, I hurt too much now to talk about it, okay?" Suspecting Moira was being facetious, Paul went home angry.

When he awoke the next morning, Saturday, he lay in bed recalling their brief conversation. Why indeed would he draw his neck in like a turtle? What was outside?

That afternoon, he pored over his scrapbooks. Reviewing his old photos in the university newspaper, he tracked changes in his posture. As a graduate student in his twenties, with his neck long and his head forward and eyes wide open, he was the picture of eager intellectual curiosity. In his thirties, when he'd achieved tenure, his head was no longer forward, but upright, as befitted an ascending pillar of academia. From his forties onward, Paul watched his head drop, year by year, into his chest.

He wondered if his vertebrae had collapsed into one another from arthritis alone, or, recalling his turtle image, if he might've unconsciously accelerated the process. Why a turtle? What happened to make him draw into his shell? Was he gradually receding from his world?

At the close of a workday, he said to Moira, "Remember when you asked me what was outside my turtle shell?"

"Yes. You seemed offended."

"Honestly, at the time, I was. I was exhausted, and hurting. But now I think what you asked was important, and I thank you for it. Do you have a couple of minutes to listen to me?"

"Sure."

Paul was surprised that as he spoke to Moira he shifted his focus from his neck and his turtle image to how demolished he'd felt when the university press rejected his book several years ago. He'd hoped that the book, as the ultimate distillation of his ideas, would establish him as a prominent contributor in his field. He recalled exactly what he'd thought the moment he learned of the rejection: *Well, I'll just shut up, then.* Or was it clam up?

As he saw a counselor over the next several weeks, the story clarified. Now Paul says, "Why should I ever withdraw? I'm not going to go into a shell the rest of my life. I have gray hair now, and that makes me an elder, so I'm going to say more of what's on my mind, not less. I'm going to take more risks, *stick my neck out.*"

Soon another publisher accepted Paul's book. As for Moira, she now attends night school to become a professional counselor. She wants eventually to get paid for what she already does so well gratis.

Like the other ways we express ourselves, our habitus, or body shape, is to some degree changeable. Try this: bring your shoulders forward as far as you can, as though you aim to touch them together in front of your chest. Now forcefully move your shoulders back, maximally protruding your breastbone, exposing your heart, so to speak. Now that you have imitated each habitus, which feels friendlier? Everyone I ask gives me the same answer. In other words, shoulders forward is one particular body language "statement," and shoulders back, another.

How do you normally—that is, when you don't think about it—carry your shoulders? A friendly configuration isn't necessarily better or worse than a protective one. Everything has its season: one situation calls for us to be defenseless, another to be guarded. As a matter of fact, a hallmark of mental health is a full repertoire of behaviors. Restriction to a single, solitary choice begs trouble; one classic definition of a "neurotic" is someone who acts the same way repeatedly yet expects different results. I recall a wonderful flyer for a men's group. It featured a photo of a Victorian beach scene in which a dozen boys in wool swimsuits grimly flexed their biceps. The caption read, TIRED OF HOLDING THAT POSE?

My friend Ken faced that kind of question. He said, "One of the things that originally attracted Peggy to me was what she called my clean-cut, can-do look, especially this square jaw of mine. After we'd been married a couple of years, though, my jaw began to hurt. I saw a series of dentists who diagnosed me every which way and recommended drugs and appliances, even surgery.

"One morning, Peggy and I were talking about it. I mentioned that I'm a healthy guy and resented having some disease in my jaw.

"Peggy said, 'Well, honey, something's going on. What if it's not a disease?'

"I said, 'If it's not a disease, then what is it?'

"She said she knew me better than anyone else, which is true, and that I clench my jaw all the time. I said no, that couldn't be so, and she said yes, it was. 'But I can't feel myself doing it,' I told her.

"We dropped it at that point, but I began to pay attention, and sure enough, she was right. I ground my teeth constantly, even made myself tired doing it. Peggy talked me into seeing a counselor, and I learned over a few weeks that all my grinding represented my mind grinding away. I didn't realize I was so constantly preoccupied by stressful thoughts.

"The counselor taught me how to relax more, and I think it's working because I don't have jaw pain for days at a time now. Peggy says I look different. No more hard, square jaw. She says I look a little softer, and she likes that, too."

Listen Carefully to His Verbal Language

We come finally to the operetta's lyrics, richly textured spoken language. All words have meanings, but some are more pictorial, conveying perspectives and sensations that abstract words cannot. When we occasionally use the wrong word, the error itself can be significant. Even silences can express meaning. And sometimes we say one thing with our mouth and another with our body, leaving our listener to judge where the truth is.

It's hardly possible to describe a bodily feeling without using a "metaphor," that legendary picture-worth-a-thousand-words. Careful attention to metaphor can reveal more of the speaker's meaning.

George visited his friend Larry, who was laid up with mid-back pain. "How goes it?" he asked.

"Terrible, thank you."

"How so?"

"Well, my back really hurts."

"Hurts like what?"

"Oh, I'd say it's a stabbing pain."

"Stabbing?"

"Yeah, something sharp here, near my spine. Like a knife. Like someone's stuck a dagger in me."

"Wow! Stuck a dagger in you?"

Larry thought about it. "Stabbed in the back, yeah, like I've been stabbed in the back." He became reflective.

"Larry," George said, "didn't you mention something like that to me last week, 'backstabbing' in your office?"

"Yeah, that's what I was just thinking about."

No one actually stabbed Larry, of course, and we can't know whether his back pain is related to office intrigue. But we do know now that Larry made some connection within his belief system between his office politics and his back pain, and that may be his first step toward healing.

Meaning regularly lurks in misstatements. My biologist friend Pete took his date, Miranda, to the beach one summer evening. Miranda asked him what caused the delightful shimmer in the breaking surf.

"Oh," he replied, "that's a red tide."

"What's a red tide?"

Anxious to impress Miranda with his knowledge—and evidently even more anxious to impress her into a mattress—Pete said, "It's bioluminescence, like what fireflies do. But here it's billions and billions of microscopic organasms . . ."

Organasms? By means of a "Freudian slip," Pete offered Miranda and the rest of us a peek into his unconscious mind. Since such "errors" occur commonly in all but the most ridiculously well guarded, the human mind must be as whimsical as it is accurate.

When you listen, don't assume that silence is necessarily unproductive. Barbara, a professional counselor, told me, "I saw a woman last week who didn't speak during the full hour we were together. I could see from her face and eye movements that she was thinking and just not ready to talk. Finally, she began to smile. It was what I'd call an ironic smile at first, but it bloomed into a grin and then a full belly laugh. I asked her what it was about, but she was so caught up in it, she waved me off. She got me laughing, too. Finally, the hour was up. She said she'd tell me about it next week. As she walked out, she turned and said, 'Thanks. I can't remember when anyone's helped me so much.'"

Occasionally, our words contradict our body language. When that happens, it's less often because we're intentionally lying than because we've lost touch with our bodies and so can only say what we guess to be true, or what we think the listener wishes to hear.

Abe appeared in the clinic for his chemotherapy. The nurse, Robin, asked him how he was doing.

"Fine," he grunted.

That's what he said, but he looked to Robin like a professional lemon taster. "Come off it, Abe," she said. "You know what *fine* means? F.I.N.E., Feelings I'm Not Expressing."

Abe laughed. "Yeah, you're right. The Feeling I'm Not Expressing is that I flat-out hate chemotherapy and I'd rather be at the racetrack."

"All right," Robin said, "at least that's a start. Now, sit down and we'll talk about it."

In listening, please keep in mind that the language of the body outpaces that of words. Our body responds almost instantly, often unthinkingly, to a situation. Our verbal responses, though, take hundreds of milliseconds. Compared to the body's language, words move like cold syrup. We choose them with more or less care, fashion them into what we hope is a comprehensible sentence, and at long last organize our lungs, vocal cords, and tongue to articulate them. So while we physically enact a meaning immediately, it usually takes us a while to speak what we mean.

It takes even longer to say with words *exactly* what we mean. Our first sentence isn't often the Whole Truth. It only approximates it, beats around the bush. But sentence by sentence, we spiral in toward precision. So expect your sick friend or relative not to speak his heart of hearts at first. He's not stalling; he simply hasn't found it yet.

Roberta asked her cousin Evvie, "So how are you doing with your emphysema?"

"Well," said Evvie, "if you really want to know, not so good."

"How's that?"

"You know how this disease cuts my breath short. I could live with that, except there are so many things I can't do."

"Like?"

"Oh, my. Well, I can't get enough breath even to get dinner together, for one thing."

"So, Evvie, what bothers you about that? I mean your neighbor Raylene comes over and cooks for you, doesn't she?"

"Sure she does, and she's an angel." Evvie paused to gather her thoughts along with her air. "But do you know what that does to me? Honey, I've been on my own since I was fourteen. I'm a self-made woman. I've always done everything for myself. Relying on somebody else just tears me up."

"Tears you up?"

"You bet it does. I'm frustrated. Sad. Angry. All those."

In that conversation Roberta encouraged Evvie to progress from her initial report of general malaise to an inventory of her discomforts, and finally to her emotional statement about feeling "torn up." Only then did she recognize aloud that her suffering was less about her emphysema than her frustration, sadness, and anger about dependency.

Both women saw then that Evvie was "torn" between her

passionate independence and her growing need for help. After considering this over the next couple of days, Evvie volunteered, "Well, Roberta, I don't think I need much help, but if helping will make Raylene and my other friends feel better, then maybe we can talk about it."

THE ILLNESS STORY AS A HOLOGRAM

An illness story, consisting as it does of the teller's mood, location, appearance, aroma, movements, story content, metaphors, slips, and pauses, is unquestionably a massive multimedia presentation. It can seem like an avalanche of information, far too much to absorb, let alone comprehend. Unless you're a trained professional, how can you take it all in?

Fortunately, although the illness story is indeed vast, it's not a jumble. In fact, it's remarkably consistent and coherent. Your sick friend or relative is telling a story with his words, to be sure, but his appearance, his gestures, and every other emanation tell exactly the same story. It doesn't drift north with a sentence and south with a gesture. *No matter where you look, you'll find a single, unified story.*

That is, we express ourselves as though we were holograms. If you can gain even a basic understanding of a hologram, your listening task will be far easier.

Of course, you've seen holograms, those three-dimensional images created by lasers. They differ from standard photographs in a crucial way. A photo records each part of its image in a specific place, while a hologram's entire image is recorded everywhere.

To conceive that, recall an image you've probably seen, a close-up of an insect's compound eye. Examining that eye's thousands of facets, you can see on each facet a reflection of whatever the insect is looking at. So it is with a hologram: everything's recorded everywhere.

Tear a photograph in half, and you'll leave yourself with half the image on each fragment. But if you tear a hologram, each piece will exhibit the entire image. Tear it into ten, twenty, a hundred pieces, and each will bear the entire image.

Something doesn't sound right here. You'd think that in reducing the hologram we'd have to lose something, and you'd be right: that's exactly what happens. Although any section carries the whole image, it does so in less detail than the unfragmented hologram. The smaller the fragment, the less resolution, the less clarity, its image will exhibit. Even though we might be assured that one one-hundredth of the original hologram still carries the whole image, its resolution will be so poor that we won't be able to recognize it.

See the body, then, as a hologram, broadcasting its illness story from every pore. With words, appearance, gestures, and aroma, we virtually spray our story out. There's nowhere we don't emit evidence, and all of it points in the same direction.

The smallest part of this broad expression, say a single word or an isolated grimace, speaks the whole story, but with minimal clarity. Add an element, and clarity improves. If you hear me groan painfully, you'll immediately know I'm more likely to be hurting or depressed than ecstatic. You'll glean more information when you notice my slumped position, and even more when you observe that I haven't shaved or brushed my teeth in days. It's starting to add up to depression, isn't it? If you are able to absorb all my expression, my entire, undivided hologram, you'll comprehend my story with perfect clarity.

If you can't achieve perfection immediately, don't worry about it. I doubt that anyone ever receives the entire package at once. Be content to get what you're getting. If all you notice is the person's words, or if the words confuse you but you sense his emotional mood and elements of his appearance, feel confident that you're comprehending the whole story through those features. With practice, you'll achieve greater resolution, appreciate his story in ever-finer detail.

Relax. Simply by being sensorily present, you'll admit this appreciable but coherent mass of information into your body. Aim less at understanding it than being open to it. My professor collected more than we students did precisely because he was relaxed. So you don't need to strain. All you need are your ears, eyes, and heart.

LISTENING WITH THE EARS, EYES, AND HEART

The Chinese written character for *listen* is compounded of those for *attention, ear, eye,* and *heart.* You've already "listened" to the illness story with your ears and eyes. To make sense of it, you'll need to listen with your heart—that is, to your own insides.

You assimilate the sick person's story, funnel the images, sounds, smells, tensions, and pressures into your brain and no doubt elsewhere, and there it all rattles around God knows how. Finally you feel its algebraic sum as just that, a feeling. That is, the sick person's story registers within you as a physical sensation.

Listening with your "heart," then, means staying tuned to precisely what you feel. You're attending carefully to the sick person and his story, and to your own consequent feelings at the same time. Compassion is literal resonance between two people, as though they were the twin tines of a tuning fork.

Harry, who was rapidly waning from lung cancer, moved in with his son Nelson. As Harry desired no heroic treatments or hospitalization, Nelson engaged the local hospice service.

Harry didn't welcome company. He was terse with visitors, even hospice nurses. He wasn't an avid reader, had no friends and few interests, and detested television. He spent his hours alone, sometimes looking out his window.

One warm Sunday afternoon, Nelson knocked on Harry's door.

"Come in."

As Nelson gently opened the door, he saw that the room was darkened and still. The windows were closed, as were the curtains. The air was humid. Nelson felt stagnation, even a sense of hopelessness.

Harry was sitting in his bed, his knees folded up against his chest. When he turned toward Nelson, his face looked pale and was stretched tightly over his skull. Nelson sat in the armchair beside the bed.

Harry said, "What?"

"Hm?"

"What is it?"

Nelson thought. "I just wanted to be with you."

"Go find something to do. You don't need to be with me."

"I said I wanted to be with you. This is what I want to do. Is it okay?" He thought he saw a smile fly quickly across his father's face. Now that the door was open, air began to circulate and Nelson felt the slightest breeze.

"All right. You're with me. Now what?"

"Nothing, I guess. I'm just with you."

Nelson looked carefully at his father. The hospice nurse had shaved Harry that morning and then, in hastily changing his pajamas, had buttoned the top wrong.

"Your pajama top's not on right," Nelson said. "Want me to fix it?"

Harry didn't hear him. "This painkiller does funny stuff to my mind," he said. "I was just lying here awake before you came in, and I thought my father was holding my hand, taking me for a walk."

Harry was eighty-three. His own father had died forty years ago. He vacantly extended his hand and opened and closed it as though grabbing at something. Nelson took Harry's hand in his, noticed the old chainsaw scar on Harry's forearm.

"Your father was taking you for a walk?"

"Yeah. I was little, maybe four or five. I guess that really happened. When my mother died she left eight kids and my father. He was helpless. All he knew was his job. He took me for a walk and told me she'd died."

Nelson noticed that Harry's eyes were wet. "I never heard you talk about that before, Dad. Do you remember how you felt then?"

Harry looked sharply at his son. "How I felt?"

"When you lost your mother."

"How do you think?" he snapped, and turned away.

"Well, if it'd been me, I guess I might've felt sad or angry or confused. I'd like to hear how it was for you."

"I hung in there."

The two men were quiet. Harry's last phrase rattled in Nelson's mind, frustrating him. His breathing suddenly became shallow, and he realized he was occupied with his own thoughts instead of being present to Harry. As he inhaled slowly, deeply, his frustration faded, and he felt once again with his father.

Harry said, "You want to know how I felt, I'll tell you. I was scared. I was scared, and I don't mind telling you. My mother was everything to me. I was much younger than my brothers and sisters, and my father was hardly ever home." He looked pleadingly at Nelson. Nelson saw a tear in his father's eye and wondered momentarily if it would drop. Harry continued, "I felt so alone. And helpless. An egg without a shell." His features softened and quickly stiffened again. "You know, you've got to be tough. It's a hard world."

"Yeah, Dad. You were tough."

"Damn straight. I hung in there." He paused. "I've got to be tough now, too. It's not easy going through this cancer business." Harry drew his hand from Nelson's and again wrapped his gaunt arms around his shins. He began to turn toward the curtains but suddenly looked into Nelson's eyes and said, "It's a lonely thing, like when my mother died. Lonely, scary."

"Yeah, it is," Nelson said. "I'm here, Dad. You're not alone now."

Harry stretched his legs out, gave Nelson his hand again. "I've been alone enough. I'm glad you're here." His face relaxed into a smile.

TO HEAL

1. Relax. Remember, the healing encounter is essentially plain old friendship.

2. Approach your sick friend or relative quietly, both to convey respect for his situation and to sense his dominant mood. Is he angry? Hopeless? Controlled? Peaceful? Needy? Confused?

3. Observe him. Notice where he is in the room and what he's doing. Notice his body: if you'd never met him, what might you presume about him from the way he looks? Notice how he holds himself, how he moves, and how he's dressed, along with other elements of his appearance.

4. Ask him about his current experience in order to elicit his illness story. "What's it like to be sick like this?" "How are your spirits?"

5. Appreciate all his language, including his metaphors, slips, and silences. Note where he's emotional in his story.

6. Note what he doesn't talk about. He has a life-threatening disease but speaks only of getting cured, or never offers a word about his wife and children.

7. Note discrepancies between his words and body language: he laughs while complaining of depression or cries while declaring that everything's fine.

8. After he's spoken, ask him questions to help him amplify his story's emotional peaks. "How did you feel when your doctor gave you that prognosis?" "Can you say more about this treatment decision you have to make?"

9. Sense your own feelings. While you're present to him, your feelings are probably similar to his. If in doubt, tell him what you feel. "I'm feeling kind of sad now. Are you?" "When I hear that, I feel angry."

SIX

SPEAKING WITH TLC

Words are so powerful, we must consider
their possible effects carefully before we speak,
and then speak only with "TLC":
truth, leanness, and compassion.

Talk low, talk slow, and don't say too much.

—John Wayne

Most people have to talk so they won't hear.

—May Sarton

WORDS CAN HEAL . . . AND WORDS CAN KILL

"Will I die from this disease?"

Cancer doctors hear that question regularly. Aiming for truth, some answer, "Yes, you'll probably die from it." But I know a doctor who tells the same truth a different way. He says, "I don't know if you'll die from it, but you'll probably live with it the rest of your life."

Until now this book has been about listening, but listening alone does not a conversation make. Sooner or later, you'll express yourself in some way. This chapter will offer guidelines for maximizing your expression's healing potential.

We can speak any thought a number of ways, and each conveys a particular feeling. In communications about sickness, one choice can emphasize hope while another wounds it. Which would you prefer, hearing that your condition carries a probability of 20 percent mortality or 80 percent survival?

If your friend or relative's immunity were compromised by the AIDS virus or a drug, you'd meticulously avoid introducing germs into her environment. Words can have a similar effect. Being sick, she's extraordinarily vulnerable to the nuances of language. Fortunately, that vulnerability ranges in both directions: whereas some words may injure her spirit, others will lift her as effectively as any pharmaceutical, and without the expense and side effects. So in order to help and to avoid harm, choose each word with care.

WHEN TO SPEAK

Before you think about what to say to your sick friend or relative, consider *when* to say it. The last thing you'd want to do is interrupt her, since that will surely interrupt her trust in you. This caution marks one difference between a healing conversation and the more popular he-said-then-she-said-then-he-said style. Just because she's quiet for the moment doesn't mean she's finished speaking. If she's using the silence to deepen her previous thought, your intrusion will impede her progress.

Therefore, you'll need to determine when it's all right for you to speak. Support groups generally honor this requirement by having members signify when they're finished speaking. In some groups, they simply say so; no one else speaks until the person has said,

"I'm finished." Other groups use a ritual object akin to the Native American "talking stick." She who holds the stick holds the floor. No one else speaks, even when she's silent. The talking stick I've used for ten years is a geode, an ordinary-looking rock cut cleanly in half to reveal its amethyst center. Having been through innumerable hands in almost two thousand meetings, it's heard much. At any rate, I suggest you devise some method to determine when it's right for you to speak, such as allowing a respectful silence and then simply asking, "Were you going to say more?"

WHAT TO SAY

Once we actually begin to speak, hopefully our concern for healing won't allow just anything to pop out of our mouths. The Greek historian Dionysius of Halicarnassus had people like me in mind when he cautioned, "Let thy speech be better than silence, or be silent." Monitoring my speaking habits, I've learned to my chagrin that there's much I say in a day that's trivial or oblique. But I believe I'm making glacial qualitative progress by routinely reflecting, *Is what I'm about to say an improvement over silence?*

Toward that end I've evolved what I call the TLC test for the healing potential of a proposed statement:

- Is it TRUE?

- Is it LEAN?

- Is it COMPASSIONATE?

TRUTH

Your sick friend or relative needs her dose of truth as regularly as she needs vitamin C. In fact, she may be starving for any shred of nailed-down certainty, since medical practice is necessarily riddled with vagueness and ambiguity. As a healer, you'll have to question continually what's true and what's only speculation, and whether your prospective statements will help her clarify her situation or simply swirl more fog around it.

My friend Mandy was lying in bed, nauseated by her medication. Her husband, Mike, asked her how she felt.

"Awful," she answered, "really awful."

"Side effects wear off," Mike said.

"What if they don't?"

Suddenly noticing a lead weight in his stomach, Mike shrugged.

Did Mike tell the truth? Will Mandy's side effects diminish? Meaning well, Mike was actually wishful-thinking aloud. He can't know whether Mandy's nausea will improve or in fact might worsen. Anyway, Mandy enjoyed no relief from their exchange. Let's listen again to learn how Mike could have handled it truthfully.

"Awful," Mandy said, "really awful."

"Hmmm. I hear you. Tell me what it's like."

"It feels like I've been on some kind of fiendish carnival ride."

"And . . ."

"Well, it feels like I've gotten off the ride and I'm lying on the ground trying to get my bearings. Everything's swimming, but maybe if I just lie here a little more . . ."

Mike's statement this time, that he heard Mandy, was true. Her recognition of his truth encouraged her to say more, and we leave Mandy now hopeful rather than punctured.

Telling the truth is an especially hefty challenge considering that our ignorance dwarfs the sum of our knowledge. If sickness is a foreign land, uncertainty is its language. Are you sure what caused your sick friend or relative's disease? Do you know for a fact that she'll die from it? Are you convinced beyond a doubt that she's made the right or wrong treatment decisions?

Although you may appreciate uncertainty's hold on this field, others who don't will present their conjectures to her as manifest truth. In addition, however anyone speaks to her, who's to say what she hears, how she interprets? Fallible human beings that we are, we'll always suffer slippage between intent and effect. Depending on an encounter's flavor, the sick person can come away feeling unrealistically buoyant or unjustifiably doomed. We probably hear enough these days about false hope; we must be equally wary of false pessimism.

Mollie, who'd had cancer for three years, had an unusually supportive family. One afternoon she phoned her cousin and close friend Earl and sobbed, "I found out I'm terminal. There's no hope."

Earl thought about it and replied, "Did the doctor tell you that?"

"Yeah, he said I was terminal."

"What does that mean, Mollie?"

"You know what terminal means. I'm going to die from it."

"Hmmm." He paused. "Does it mean you're dying now?"

"No, silly, I'm not dying now."

"Do you have some idea when you're going to die, then?"

"Of course not."

"Then, Mollie: what's changed? What do you know now besides that you have cancer and that one day you'll die?"

In your conversations with sick people, speculation—including medical statistics and words like *terminal*—will undoubtedly arise. Let's explore this issue so you'll be in a better position to help them sort the theoretical from the real.

Is Mollie truly terminal? If "terminal" means she'll eventually die, then we're all terminal. Does "terminal" mean she'll die sooner rather than later, or only that she's likely to? How likely? What is "sooner"? As you've no doubt guessed, I've abandoned that word and so have numerous other physicians. It's useless at best and voodoo at worst. If Mollie feels she's not dying now, how can it serve anyone to convince her that she is?

The tendencies, probabilities, and statistics that help guide doctors—and consequently patients and their caregivers—are only what they claim to be, likelihoods. They're medically useful, but when taken as solid predictions they can be hazardous.

My friend Ed, who's been treated for malignant melanoma the past two years, was given ever-changing odds. He says, "When he diagnosed me, my doc said that based on statistics, I probably wouldn't be around more than six months.

"Now, I've never been all that interested in statistics. To my mind, they predict with great precision which way the wind *might* blow. But what the doc said really crushed my wife. For a week, she felt sicker than I did.

"When I lived past six months, the doc found new numbers. He told us I had a 20 percent chance of living another year. Well, that put my wife in bed, crying for four days. Neither of us needs that kind of grief. My year's passed now. I let my doc know I don't want to hear any more numbers. There are only two statistics that interest me these days, 100 percent and zero: either I'm here or I ain't."

The best we doctors can do is to guess intelligently what caused someone's sickness; we can't know for sure. Nor can we know how she'll respond to treatment or when or how she'll die.

Nonmedical people don't generally appreciate medicine's inevitable ambiguities. Indeed, the news media's relentless touting of medical progress primes them to assume certainty where it isn't, and that can lead to trouble.

My friend Marika told me, "When my husband, Max, got diagnosed with multiple sclerosis twenty years ago, the doctor said the disease would move rapidly and Max would probably be dead in five years. We'd been raised to have total confidence in doctors' pronouncements. We didn't know then that every prediction has built-in leeway. So we put our plans to have kids on hold.

"As time went on, though, Max remained fairly stable. He had flares now and then, and it got to the point he needed to walk with a cane, but we still expected the disease to overtake him. Whenever he'd raise the question of kids, I'd remind him of his prognosis as gently as I could.

"His doctor died two years ago, and Max began to see a new one. This one said Max's MS was a less vicious type than was recognized when we'd first been told. I guess after eighteen years we'd already figured that out, but if we'd initially known how slowly the disease might move, we'd have done differently, probably had kids. It grieves me that we didn't. I know now that doctors can't read the future, but I didn't know it then."

Once you insist on representing only what you know to be true as the truth, you'll find not only that you speak less, but that a substantial amount of your healing work will lie in helping sick people tease their needle of truth from their haystack of speculation. And a haystack it is, since our particular universe is permeated, if not entirely characterized, by uncertainty.

Some degree of fuzziness—an indeterminate portion, at that—surrounds even the "hardest" sciences. The late Richard Feynman, who received the Nobel Prize in physics in 1965, wrote in his last book, *The Pleasure of Finding Things Out:*

. . . the real value of science may lie in uncertainty.

The scientist has a lot of experience with ignorance and doubt and uncertainty, and this experience is very important. Scientific knowledge is a body of statements of varying degrees of certainty—about some of them we are mostly unsure, some are nearly certain, none are *absolutely* certain. We scientists are used to this, and we take it for granted that it is perfectly consistent to be unsure, that it is possible to live and not to know. But I don't know whether everyone realizes that this is true.[1]

As a scientist, I have to agree with Dr. Feynman that no one knows much about anything with absolute certainty. In fact, I'm aware of only four things we can know about a sick person and she can know about herself.

• We know she's sick.

• We know she'll die: sick or not, she's as mortal as anyone else.

• We know she's alive now.

• We know our feelings as we relate to her.

To the degree we adhere to these "knowabilities," we're telling the truth. But it's difficult to build our end of the conversation from these alone. So feel free to succumb to the natural temptation to speculate. Just be aware that you're doing so, and lower your healing expectations during that time.

If our own feelings make up one category of truth, how appropriate is it to express them to the sick person? Caregivers frequently confide in me their worry that they'll alarm or depress the sick person if they cry in front of her. I tell them that while they accurately see emotion as contagious, I've never seen a caregiver's emotion damage the sick person, and I've often seen it help. At least it clears the air, a valuable service since we can't effectively hide our emotion anyway. Unusually sensitive to others, the sick person has probably already sensed our body language and is even aware that part of what we feel is our reticence to express it. A conspiracy not to discuss this, then, amounts to a metaphorical rhino stomping through the room, wreaking havoc while the human beings present pretend they don't see it. In addition, the sick person will wonder what else we're withholding from her, and her trust in us will decline.

Besides, our feelings are as valid as hers. As you know, sickness radiates suffering outward into relatives and friends. So drop the notion that she's the "patient" and we're the "healer," since we're both hurting and we're both treatable. I've heard this perspective described as the We're-all-bozos-on-this-bus school of healing. A potent but often ignored treatment is helping others: our pain might be her opportunity.

A few years ago, while I was facilitating a cancer support group, a nurse interrupted to tell me I had an important phone call. It was my wife, who told me my father had just died. Although I'd been expecting it, it was still a shock. After I hung up, I sat alone quietly for ten minutes. During that time, the nurse informed the group what had happened. I felt crushed but decided to finish the meeting. I returned and sat down. When I tried to speak, no words emerged. All I could do was cry. The group's members, none short of major problems themselves, surrounded and held me. Only if I become a poet will I be able to describe my appreciation. The following week the group talked about how healed they'd felt as they healed someone else.

Veracity is one aspect of truth in healing speech, and another is relevancy: some truths simply aren't pertinent to the conversation at hand. Within a healing encounter, unless what we choose to say addresses that sick person's immediate suffering, it's unhelpful.

Rebecca is a professional pianist who developed rheumatoid arthritis in her hands. Though she was maximally medicated, her joints continued to swell, affecting her piano technique. One afternoon she and her close friend Ida went out for tea.

"I don't know how much longer I can perform," she told Ida.

Ida replied, "My mother had rheumatoid arthritis, too, you know. She'd dip her hands in hot melted wax and let it cool and then she'd peel the wax off, and it always made a big difference."

Let's ignore for the moment that Ida was trying to fix Rebecca and dissect the transaction a little differently. Even though what Ida said was true, that her mother had indeed benefited from hot wax treatment, her recommendation was irrelevant to the suffering Rebecca had only begun to articulate. In addressing the physical disease, even with truth, Ida departed from Rebecca's feelings—probably because her friend's pain was beginning to hurt her, Ida—and pushed instead for a physical fix.

LEANNESS

How much truth should we say? If we say too little, we'll fail to express what we mean, and if we say too much, the listener will be overwhelmed and tune out. I recommend erring on the side of brevity, since what the sick person says will generally promote her healing more effectively than anything we say.

To see how excess truth can generate distress, *unheal,* the next time you're in a library, find the standard *Physician's Desk Reference.* The PDR lists every American pharmaceutical, its chemistry, indications for use, and so on. Look up the side effects of a few common drugs. I guarantee you'll be alarmed by their quantity and occasionally horrendous quality. Your doctor wisely avoids reading you the whole list, and not because she wishes to withhold the truth from you. The reality is that every drug poses a few common side effects and a huge spread of rare ones, so a complete reading would frighten more than educate.

My friend Zelda glimpsed this issue's core when her four-year-old daughter, Amy, asked her, "Mommy, where did I come from?"

Zelda replied, "Well, honey, sit down here with me and I'll tell you. Uh, you know how Daddy looks like he does and I look like I do, how women and men are built differently? Well . . ."

"Mommy, I was playing with Jessica and she said she came from Milwaukee. Where did I come from?"

So it was that Zelda learned to determine exactly what sort of information Amy sought before answering her. We can't know what's demanded of us unless we ask.

Beyond its potential to anguish, too much talk can actually squelch a relationship. My friend Fred told me, "After I was diagnosed with prostate cancer, a social worker gave me a phone number. She said to call this guy Archie, since he'd had pretty much the same kind of cancer I have. I phoned him, we chatted awhile, and I told him I needed more information.

"If he'd allowed me to get another word in, I would've explained that I wanted to find out where I could sit down with a bunch of guys who've been through prostate cancer and hear their experiences. That's the kind of information I wanted.

"But I guess Archie loves to talk. He told me about every prostate cancer book and magazine, every Web site, the names and phone numbers of the country's top urologists, and on and on. Frankly, he gave me a headache, and I guess I was just too polite to stop him. I looked forward to hanging up, and I didn't even write down what he told me."

Do people like Archie just love to talk, or is there something more profound afoot? Bill, who was hospitalized for complications of his kidney cancer, told me, "Couple of days ago my golfing buddy Vic dropped in to see me. He asked me how I was, and I said something like 'Getting along.' Then he told me about the people he's known who've had cancer. This one saw some super surgeon, that one went to a Chinese clinic. And wouldn't you know it, every damn one of them got cured. When he ran out of miracles, he said, 'Hey, good to see you, amigo. Great you're doing so well,' and he left.

"I kept thinking about that visit. I'll bet I could've left a photo of me in bed and walked out, and he would've kept talking. He went home with no idea how I was doing.

"Yesterday he visited again. I just came out and asked him about that. I said, 'I'm glad to see you, Vic, but why do you feel like you have to keep talking, telling me about all those cures?'

"He got really quiet then. He looked down at the floor, and when he finally answered me he was a different man. He said, 'Bill, the fact is I'm plenty afraid for you. I can't bring myself to even imagine you getting sicker or dying. All I want to think about is playing golf with you again, so I make myself focus on cures.'

"Well, that certainly gave me pause. I can count on the fingers of one hand how many times anyone's ever spoken that honestly with me, and I told him so. We went on to have a really close conversation."

My friend Andy, who happens to be a doctor, had an experience similar to Bill's. He told me, "When I had an MRI of my head, I waited while the film developed, and the radiologist invited me to look at the pictures with him.

"He found a tumor in my brain. It was only the size of a pea, but that little shadow instantly evicted me from my life. I felt like I was in a train speeding out of the station, being kidnapped from my family and friends, my practice, everything.

"I just sat there, stunned. I realized after some time that the radiologist was speaking to me. He was saying something about treatment, surgery, radiation—I'm not sure, since I couldn't really hear him. It was like we were both underwater. He was telling me words, but his eyes said something else. His eyes said fear. I realized he probably saw himself in me, and it scared him. We're both doctors about the same age, with families: this could have been him as easily as me.

"He was pumping out all that talk to insulate himself. I don't hold that against him. He's a good doctor, a decent man. He has a right to be frightened. I would've felt better, though, if he'd just said to me, 'You know, Andy, this scares the hell out of me.' Saying that would've been true, and as a matter of fact it would've been all I needed to hear then. We didn't both have brain tumors, but we were both scared, so I'd have felt at least like I wasn't alone in my fear."

Another way to speak excessively is to shout. My friend Jim was hospitalized to have his diabetes regulated. He told me, "I actually had a good time in the hospital. My visitors and the doctors and staff treated me wonderfully except for one woman from my office. She wasn't nasty to me, just spoke loud, like I was hard of hearing. She didn't look me in the eye, either. She'd never acted that way in the office, but at my bedside she sounded like she was calling to me from thirty feet away.

"Maybe she wished she *was* thirty feet away. I know she cares about me, but maybe she doesn't have a lot of experience visiting sick people. Could be it scares her. At any rate, I didn't have the energy to go into it with her then, to be her counselor or whatever. It was my turn to be sick. But when I get back to work, I'd like to take her out to lunch and ask her about it."

COMPASSION

To be compassionate is ideally to feel what the sick person feels, and so to treat her kindly. That means telling her—leanly, of course—the truth that we believe will help her feel better at this moment.

I once worked in an emergency department alongside an older licensed vocational nurse named Bernice. Lower on the skills ladder than a registered nurse, Bernice couldn't insert intravenous lines or give injections, but her particular talent was invaluable.

Late one night an ambulance delivered a young man who'd broken both arms and both legs in a motorcycle accident. The nursing team and I pressed around him, working feverishly, but we parted for Bernice.

She looked down at the pale and frightened man, appraised his condition, and with a soft smile said, "Honey, you're a mess. You're in rough shape, but we're gonna do our best with you." She touched his cheek and beamed at him, and despite his injuries, he smiled.

If it ever seems that the most compassionate thing you can say isn't exactly true, consider stretching your notion of truth. Compassion never entails lying but sometimes requires honestly seeing a wider reality, a process that will heal you as much as it does the other person.

My friend Sue said, "Whenever I'd visit my father in his Alzheimer's care home, I left troubled. I couldn't understand why every visit bothered me until I made it a point to watch closely, and then I learned what it was.

"It began when he asked me, 'Am I home now?'

"Naturally, I told him the truth each time. I'd say, 'No, Dad, you're not. You're in a place where people can take good care of you.' Then he'd look glum the rest of my visit. I figured, sure, I could humor him and tell him he was home, but that wouldn't have been true.

"The thing was, though, that they really did take good care of him there. They were loving, and certainly gave him more attention than I could've. I started thinking, well, why didn't I call that place his home?

"So the next time he asked, 'Am I home now?' I said, 'Yes, Dad, you are,' and you should've seen him brighten up. Maybe he wanted reassurance that he'd continue to stay there, I don't know. In any case, when I softened around what the actual truth was, we both felt better."

Estelle's cancer moved into her vertebrae and eventually damaged her spinal cord, leaving her quadriplegic. Her sister Freddie had her admitted to a skilled nursing facility. Once Estelle was moved in, her cancer inexplicably came to an apparent halt. Having been psychologically primed to die, Estelle became frustrated over the next two months with her now unpredictable course.

When Freddie visited Estelle one morning, she saw a dark frown on her face. "What's up, Estelle?"

"This cancer."

"What about it?"

"It comes, it goes. It's confusing."

"Confusing? How?"

Estelle thought. "Well, what's going on? Am I living or dying?"

"Funny you mention it. I've been wondering that for a while, too."

"And your conclusions . . . ?"

"Without a doubt, you're living."

Estelle's frown grew. "Living? What kind of a life is this?"

"I've thought of that, too. I guess it's yours, Estelle, as hard as it is. I wouldn't be wild about it, either, but this is your life, right here. I can't get around that."

"So maybe this is a lifestyle, right?" Nodding, Estelle changed her frown to a questioning look.

Over the next month, Estelle began to insist on turning herself in bed rather than relying on nurses. Pulling on her overhead trapeze with the feeble arm strength left to her, she'd take an hour to turn and then proudly announce, "Hell of a lifestyle, but what the hell, it's mine."

Our capacity for compassion depends on sensitivity to our own suffering. The principle of the "wounded healer," which permeates every culture, suggests that it's those who have suffered who heal others best. When I was a young doctor and hadn't been long in the real world—a stranger to personal suffering—I saw patients mainly as intellectual problems for me to solve. I didn't resonate with their suffering because I hadn't the matrix of my own upon which to hang it.

Now that I've sampled my share, I act differently with sick people. As we age, we accumulate suffering as surely as we gather wrinkles, so at least we have the opportunity, when listening to a

sick person's illness story, to recall our own suffering and so resonate with her. Suddenly, she's no longer separate from us but
rather shares our skin, as though we've expanded our selfhood to
include her. Indeed, that's compassion's technology.

To the extent we avoid our own suffering, we'll fail to heal
ourselves, and consequently those we contact. Yet we naturally
resist sensing our own suffering, and not only because it's an un-
pleasant feeling. To suffer in front of another shatters the illu-
sion of our invulnerability. To those of us who prefer to
romanticize our healing role by appearing impeccably hearty
and in control, vulnerability is anathema.

This challenge can especially vex males. I have some feeling for
this since I was raised as a male. I was implicitly encouraged to be
strong and silent, keep a stiff upper lip, hide all weakness. That
direction changed radically for me once I realized that expressing
my emotions honestly wasn't displaying a defect. Indeed, considering the requisite effort of will, it was an act of courage.

TOUCH

Contact is a touchy issue, not to be taken lightly.

When we touch someone appropriately, it can help heal her.
Done otherwise, it can harm.

Numerous studies of human beings and other mammals
show that all else being equal, babies thrive when they're lovingly
handled. Touch seems to transfer emotional energy, like pressing
a wet sponge to a dry one. By hugging a crying child, we take on
a share of her misery, literally lighten her load. By holding a
feeble sick person's hand, we transfuse her spirit with a dose of
our vigor or faith.

Touch isn't always a benevolent transfer. We touch saints and
celebrities to cherish their energy, even though aware that by

doing so we might deplete them. Sometimes with touch we manipulate others, or reinforce a pecking order. Be honest: whom are you more likely to backslap, your boss or your employee?

An emotional calculus would measure an encounter's healing by the degree both parties enjoy it. A genuine healing contact leaves you and your sick friend or relative feeling better, whether you gave or received emotional energy.

Even though we generally crave being touched and appreciate its healing benefits when we're sick, we can resist it occasionally from a need for solitude or modesty. At these times, contact is stressfully intrusive and so will retard healing. In other words, there are times to touch and times not to touch; it's important that we determine what's needed at the moment.

This demands our flexibility, since we know we'll find ourselves in situations where we're drawn strongly to touch or not touch. You can begin to discern and hopefully extend your flexibility by recognizing your own feelings about being touched. I'm not concerned with what your feelings are. I ask you to review them only in order to recognize them, since *you'll heal most effectively when your behavior flows from you naturally.*

So how do you feel about being touched? In what situations do you prefer it and avoid it? Is it generally more important to you to contact sick people physically or to keep some space between you? If you enjoy touching others, ask yourself why. Does contact bring you closer to them? Does it ever give you a feeling of eroticism or power? Do you believe the "laying on of hands" is a healing treatment? If so, is your touch a clinical act or more an expression of your relationship?

And then there's age. In our culture, the young generally are more comfortable with touching than our oldest generation is. When is it okay for you to touch a child, particularly someone else's child? And how, and where, to touch? What about children of the opposite gender?

Touch is, of course, closely related to sexuality. Contact between women and men inevitably triggers some element, however subtle, of romance, seduction, power, harassment, or rejection. Endemic homophobia renders contact between men uniquely thorny. I don't care how liberated you are: most men still like putting one urinal between them and the next guy.

Considering all this, I suggest you first observe your use of touch outside healing encounters. Learn what touching or not touching means to you. Notice when you enjoy being touched and when you avoid or resent it. It's only through respect for touch's potency that we'll effect healing when we caress a head or lay our hand on a shoulder—or decline to do so.

My friend Marnie has had lymphoma for five years. A year ago, her oncologist told her it was no longer responding to medication, that there was nothing more he could do for her except ease her symptoms.

"It was strange hearing that because I actually felt well," Marnie said. "I'd planned to do plenty of alternative treatments anyway, and it seemed the doctor's news freed me to start on that path. In other words, despite what he told me, I was spiritually in good shape.

"But my husband was comparatively fragile. I dreaded passing the news on to him. His mother had died just a month before, and he'd only begun to grieve. So I didn't want the doctor to tell him about me. I wanted to tell him myself, and in the gentlest way I could.

"I sat him down, and right away I knew he suspected the worst. His jaw began to tremble. So before I said anything, I took his hand. I put my other arm around him and squeezed him. He was in my arms, being cared for. Then I told him. I also told him I felt well and wasn't about to give up.

"After we'd both cried awhile, he said, 'Well, I guess that's what the doctor said, but you're still here, and stronger still. Marnie, you're an inspiration.'"

Sonja's daughter Randy was born with cystic fibrosis and was hospitalized dozens of times. Though she'd been affectionate as a young child, Randy gradually began to resist her mother's contact. It pained Sonja when Randy recoiled from her hugs.

"What is it?" Sonja demanded. "What's wrong?"

"Nothing," Randy snapped. "I just don't like people to touch me."

Sonja assumed this was a "phase" through which Randy would pass, so she continued to press her affections while hoping Randy would change.

One day, when Sonja came to visit her in the hospital and bent to kiss her, an exasperated fifteen-year-old Randy said, "Mom, when are you ever going to accept who I am?"

That caught Sonja's attention. Thinking about it later, she realized her own thwarted need had come to sour their relationship. She consciously decided to honor Randy's preference and to do so sincerely, without resentment. She knew this wouldn't be easy but knew as well that the stakes were high.

The next evening she entered Randy's room and demurely sat at her bedside. She was as loving and concerned as ever, but during her stay kept her hands to herself and never even leaned toward her daughter. When she said goodnight and turned to walk out, she noticed that Randy looked slightly confused.

Sonja returned the next morning. As on her previous visit, she greeted Randy verbally and sat without attempting to touch her.

"Mom," Randy inquired, "you've changed something, haven't you?"

"Yes, I have. How do you feel about it?"

A tear welled in Randy's eye. "Mom, I think you're beginning to see who I am. Thanks."

Conversations like these are qualitatively unusual. They differ from their ordinary, social cousins in pace and depth, and in addition they change both parties. Your openness and acceptance, your flexibility, and your lean and compassionate use of spoken truth will help transform your sick friend or relative's consciousness, and you can expect to change as well. You'll discover you've both moved beyond your accustomed limits. Because of its transformative nature, you might come to regard a healing conversation as special indeed, even sacred. Who knows the depths such an encounter can realize, the results that might accrue? Indeed, there may be no end to healing.

TO HEAL

1. Don't interrupt. If you're unsure whether your sick friend or relative is finished speaking, ask in order to be sure. "Were you going to say more?"

2. Think before speaking. Consider whether your words will exceed the benefit of silence. Do you really need to say, "Well, if you're going to get cancer, yours is the kind to get," or would it be better to say nothing?

3. *Before answering her question, determine what she really seeks and, if possible, help her answer it herself.* When she asks, "Do you think I should take the treatment my doctor recommends?" is she simply asking for your feelings about her treatment or is she looking for someone to decide for her? You can say, "I'm honestly not sure what you should do. What route do you feel most comfortable with?"

4. *Say what you know to be true.* Not true: "I know you're going to be cured of this." True: "I know your diagnosis is serious, and I also know that some people live with it." Admit what you don't know, label your speculations as such, and express your own feelings.

5. *Speak leanly,* saying just enough to express your truth but not so much that your listener is overwhelmed or your verbiage separates the two of you.

6. *Speak with compassion,* the kindest intent. Instead of saying only, "Yes, you *are* a burden," consider, "Yes, you are needy now, and I'll be needy sometime, too."

7. *Don't routinely touch or avoid touching.* Weigh each opportunity as cautiously as you do each word.

SEVEN

WELCOMING MYSTERY

> *Sickness can be an opportunity for profound,*
> *even transformative, growth.*

The most beautiful experience we can have is the mysterious. It is the fundamental emotion which stands at the cradle of true art and true science.

—Albert Einstein

I sit at the table of unknowing and invite you to join me there.

—Dalai Lama

HEALING BEYOND HEALING

There's no limit to healing. Equanimity is a wonderful attainment, but sometimes it's only an existential hors d'oeuvre that precedes the delicious entrée, personal transformation.

My friend Ramona said, "The moment my doctor told me I had lymphoma, I had a very disturbing thought: *Ah, a way out.*

"Things weren't going well long before my diagnosis. I'd always accommodated people too much, I think, but my husband and teenagers squeezed that for all it was worth. They treated me like a doormat. Ramona, cook dinner. When will you do the laundry? Mom, clean my room. I hated my life. So when the lymphoma came, it seemed like a weird kind of gift. It really was a way out. Now my family will treat me better because I'm sick, I thought, and if they don't, I'll die anyway. However Gary and the kids act, I'll win.

"But I hadn't figured on chemotherapy putting me into remission. Of course, I was happy about my remission, but a little disappointed too. Here I was, still alive and with my family still treating me terribly. The remission ruined my plans.

"So I found myself in this strange, totally unexpected situation. I began to take time just to sit with that, wonder what it was about. For days at a time, I hardly said a word. Gary thought I was depressed. He wanted to take me to the doctor. I told him I wasn't, that I was just being quiet.

"You wouldn't think that having your death sentence commuted would be scary, but it was. When I was dying, there was nothing I needed to do. The disease would take charge and all I'd need to do was ride along. But now, apparently, I was sentenced to life. If I wasn't to be continually miserable, I came to realize, I'd have to change my life, and no one could do that but me.

"I don't know where I came up with the idea, but I did a private little ceremony one afternoon when I was home alone. I found a photo of myself that I hated. I looked so wimpy in it. The longer I sat and looked at it, the angrier I got. Finally I told it, 'Adios, girl, you're out of here.' And then I burned it.

"That night, when Gary came home and whined that dinner wasn't ready, I snapped at him. 'Make it yourself,' I said, and I stalked out of the room. To put it mildly, he was taken aback. Maybe he still thought I was depressed, or that the chemo had damaged my brain.

"I stewed by myself until something inside me burst. Gary and the kids were eating peanut butter and jelly sandwiches in the kitchen. I barged in and said, 'You're looking at the new me.' I actually screamed it. I wasn't used to being angry, and I think it scared them. I told them from then on I was no longer their servant. I had my own life. They'd have to take turns cooking, washing dishes, doing the laundry. 'The old Ramona's dead and gone,' I said. 'Find a way to get along without her!'

"That was a rough night. The next day, though, I was able to talk without screaming. But I stayed firm. I told them my lymphoma was a loud and clear message that I couldn't go on like I had been. I suggested they pretend that the old Ramona had died and was replaced by a strong woman with her own life. Take it or leave it.

"That was four years ago. They took it, and actually did pretty well with it. They're more independent now, and I think we're all closer for that. They're pretty good cooks, too. I recently started taking my turn, but no more than my turn. I spend more time away from home now, taking classes and doing things I like, learning more who I am. I love this life."

Gary, Ramona's husband, told the story from his perspective. "When Ramona screamed at me and the kids in the kitchen that night, she scared us to death. We thought she'd gone crazy. I'd always seen us as a normal, typical family. I was comfortable with the way we'd been doing things, and now, suddenly, Ramona threw a wrench into the works. That hurt. I didn't know where it'd lead. All I wanted was our old life back.

"But Ramona was sick, so the kids and I talked about it and

gave her some slack. We organized the housework to take it off her hands for a while. That 'a while' dragged out, though, and after a few months it became routine.

"Ramona spent more time with her friends and in classes. When she was home, I began to notice a change in her: she really had become a stronger person. She was happier, too, and I felt good about that. I wonder now if over the years we'd slipped into unhealthy family habits.

"She's stayed in remission. These days, when she tells me anything about herself, I really listen. I don't assume she's depressed or crazy or abnormal at all. Matter of fact, because of what she's been through I think she's that much wiser, and that she can teach me a few things."

ENTERING MYSTERY

When Ramona first considered what her remission meant to her, she found a blitz of uncertainties. Who was she now? What if her family found her outbursts intolerable? Was she sliding into insanity? She didn't try to solve these riddles, only got quiet and lived with them, and finally, as though some invisible teletype were printing directions for her, she began to find her way.

Passively remaining with her riddles couldn't have been easy for her. Hardly anyone's eager to sit still when he has crucial decisions to make. You've read repeatedly in this book about the uncertainties that necessarily pervade sickness and healing, and probably know from your own experience the discomforts they can generate. You might prefer, then, that I reassure you about what's known rather than flaunt what isn't. But, no, I'd rather continue exploring uncertainty itself, since it's actually a path toward deeper healing.

We're talking about mystery, the intersection of suffering's tumult and healing's equanimity, the whirlwind from out of which God spoke to Job. I find poetic justice in the notion that the very center of suffering holds clues to its alleviation.

The word *mystery* comes from the Greek *myein*, "to close, be shut." A mystery's contents are hidden from our ordinary senses. For healing purposes, let's view mystery a little differently than we ordinarily do—not as a closed box to be opened or a puzzle we can solve or not solve, but as a realm we can inhabit.

When we do enter it, the first thing we notice is its darkness. That shouldn't surprise us. As the domain of all unknowns, mystery is obscurity beyond anything we can conceive. Yet we're drawn to it anyway, probably by our relentless faith that this universe operates by some sort of rhyme and reason.

Our faith isn't blind faith. The entire history of science amounts to a rather fruitful search for pattern within the apparently random. Indeed, scientists so consistently detect pattern that some naturally wonder whether there are *patterns of patterns*, and a few surmise that there's some ultimate pattern encompassing all others. Thus Albert Einstein's oft-quoted comment, "I want to know God's thoughts. The rest is details."

Spiritual traditions everywhere recognize this master pattern, this mystery of mysteries, calling it variously the Law, the Way, the Tao, dharma, cosmic consciousness, and so on. They agree that while we're too limited to know it directly, we're free to sense its immanence and conform ourselves to it.

They agree as well that since we have no more influence over it than an ant has over the moon's orbit, we certainly can't demand anything of it. We can't make it reveal its wisdom to us. All we can do is to enter and occupy it mindfully, which is to say surrender ourselves to a state of grace. Then, if it's to reveal something to us, it will.

WHY ME?

The voyage into mystery begins when we ask some version of "Why me?" Upon falling seriously sick, we naturally shift our focus from daily trivia toward larger concerns. Whereas before diagnosis we'd been content to consider nothing more profound than what time to pick up the dry cleaning, today we can't avoid the grandest possible questions. Why am I sick in this particular way? Why now? Why me and not someone else? Why do knaves thrive while the good die young? Is the universe random and absurd, or, if I look, might I find meaning, justice, mercy?

How we begin the search—how we ask our question—is crucial. My friend Bonnie developed insulin-dependent diabetes. It destroyed her and her husband, Lee, for weeks, but especially her. She was used to nonstop moving, doing, accomplishing, and now she suddenly had to excuse herself several times a day, sit down and jab her finger, test her blood sugar, and give herself an insulin injection.

Nor was that the only disruption. She was stymied everywhere, even when she shopped for food. She couldn't toss things into her cart on the run as she'd always done. Instead, she had to stop and read every item's label and think about calories and exchanges.

She resented diabetes for wrecking her life. "Why me?" she constantly asked. "Why me?"

Eventually Lee tired of hearing that, so he asked Bonnie what she meant by it.

She said, "Well, why did I get diabetes? What was it about me? My genes? Something I ate? A toxin?"

Bonnie was determined to find the cause. She read books, downloaded reams of information from the Internet. She turned up clues here and there but was never able to nail anything down. Rather than feeling she was getting closer to a useful answer, she admitted she was gradually becoming more confused.

Her question so consumed her, though, that Lee encouraged her to stick with it but find some way to ask it more productively. Bonnie began to tilt it more toward "What's going to happen to me? What'll this do to my future?" Unfortunately, most of the answers she found to these questions were disappointing lists of complications in dreadful detail. That course only frightened her.

Lee realized that Bonnie's first strategy was rooted in her past, searching for the cause, and her second involved her future, what might happen to her. The one view she hadn't tried was of the present, so he asked her what "Why me?" meant to her right now.

Bonnie sat down and just reflected on what she felt at that moment. When she stayed with that, answers came and she began to make progress. She saw something that had been perfectly obvious to Lee, but not to her because she hadn't wanted to see it—that diabetes just plain slowed her down.

Looking at her life from this new, slow lane, she saw that it wasn't all bad. She realized that when she stopped to test her blood, she was examining her life, too. During those few minutes, she reflected on where she was and what she was doing.

She gradually saw opportunities she'd never noticed from her characteristic fast track. She imagined renovating her job. She told her boss, and he supported her ideas. After making those changes, she found she stayed relaxed at work while actually accomplishing more.

Now Bonnie's had diabetes for three years. Lee says he wouldn't have wished it on her, but it's changed her in some beneficial ways, mainly helped her to see her life more clearly and find ways to get what she wants.

"That hasn't been lost on me, either," he says. "By acting as she did, she showed me how to take charge of my own life, and I didn't even have to get sick to do it."

The past is no more and the future's a hypothesis. Bonnie's mystery exists only in this moment. By shifting her "Why me?" focus toward the present, Bonnie finally entered her mystery. It revealed to her that her suffering lay principally in the disease's brakes on her accustomed pace. She first saw how the slower rate dented her style. As she remained in her mystery, kept watching, it continued to unfold. It showed her possibilities nested in those dents, and she gradually acted to make some of them real. Bonnie attained relative serenity about her disease—and that might have been healing enough—but engagement with her mystery impelled her further. She progressed steadily from initial devastation to survival to healing to a state of increasing fulfillment.

In my experience, stories like Bonnie's are by no means rare, yet they haven't entirely captured our thinking. We don't normally study people like Bonnie to learn how they adapt to their disease, let alone how some of them use it as a springboard toward a better life. We do, however, get curious when diseases inexplicably vanish. Studies of cancer patients who've had what we call spontaneous remissions generally report these people to be "weller than well," as though something within their sickness experience boosted them beyond their prediagnostic wellness level. When asked why this happened, they, the patients, uniformly respond that it wasn't a spontaneous process at all but a result of deliberate action. They mean many things by this, including the wishes of others, changes in their own perceptions, and divine intervention. But whatever the source of "weller than well," we must admit that how it comes about is outside our ordinary perspective.

SPIRITUALITY

Healing in the degree experienced by Bonnie and others like her is a spiritual process. It might be reasonable to call it transformational, since it substantially changes the person, but I believe it's most honest to label it spiritual because it edges toward absolutes: a few people become even weller than "weller than well." In fact, we don't know this phenomenon's ultimate limits.

I use the word *spirituality* cautiously since it can be as troublesome a word as *love*. We too easily connect it with religion, ghosts, angels, piety, and séances. I confess that in the days when I was a harder-nosed scientist than I am now, I thought of spirituality as something between irrelevancy and airheadedness. Spirituality's place in organized religion looks positive or negative to us depending on whether the version we encountered in childhood helped edify us or, conversely, twist us. In fact, few other words raise the mass of flak that *spiritual* does.

By spirituality I mean something so simple it's hopefully ecumenical: *expansion of self-image.* A wider sense of self is a larger tool kit for life: a hammer and saw build a better home than a hammer alone.

As we expand self-image, realize our greater complexity, we discover a richer range of perception and consequently of behavior. Viewing the world from a single set of eyes yields only one vision, whereas additional perspectives allow just that, additional perspective. If I can sense a given event, such as my sickness, from several angles, I'll comprehend it in greater depth and detail. Then I'll see possibilities invisible to a more cursory examination and so enjoy greater latitude of response.

My friend Jim, bothered by increasing back and abdominal pain, became jaundiced. Already believing his condition to be serious, he wasn't entirely surprised when his doctor told him he had pancreatic cancer. As kindly as he could, the doctor added that Jim's tumor type was usually resistant to treatment. All he could do, he said, was to relieve Jim's symptoms.

Jim was a plumber with ardent interests outside his work. In his youth he'd had a successful band, and he still played music regularly with his friends. He was also a respected member of a close-knit, meditation-oriented community.

Jim's hospital nurses were amazed at the quantity of visitors this bachelor enjoyed. They filled his room, and still more stood in line in the corridor to see him. They transformed every surface into an altar. Along with Jim, they understood death to be sad and inconvenient, but in its inevitability normal, too. They believed this life was undeniably meaningful, and at the same time only one of many incarnations.

A few days before Jim died, his musician friends gathered around his bed and serenaded him until he requested his own guitar so he could join them. Leaving, one told him, "I'll be gone over the weekend, so I'm not sure I'll see you again."

Jim chuckled. "Oh yes, you will. Next time around."

The broader I consider myself to be, the more I can afford to lose when I get sick or disabled. (I say "when," not "if," because short of sudden, unexpected death, we're all certain to lose flesh and function.) If I see myself only as a male, loss of my sexuality will summarily flatten me. But if I see myself as a male and a middle-aged person and a chef and a fisherman, I'll be less distressed when one identity wanes.

Not everyone achieves this sort of stretch. I heard about William, a traveling salesman. Divorced and with no children, he found that life on the road was right for him. In fact, he so sparkled at it that he barely missed having close friends and hobbies. During one of his trips, he suffered a heart attack in a hotel room. After two weeks of hospitalization he returned home and recovered satisfactorily, but his supervisor feared returning him to his route.

Wounded, William protested, "But it's what I do. It's who I am."

His supervisor stood firm: upon William's return to work, he'd have a desk job or nothing. William watched television and went for short walks but remained resentful, despondent, and unable to regain his driving force. A month after being laid off, he suffered a second heart attack, which proved fatal.

There's no way to know in advance who will and who won't grow spiritually, into deeper healing.

When it was apparent that eighty-five-year-old Aaron was rapidly succumbing to several concurrent diseases, his niece Yvonne moved him from the hospital into a nursing home. There, at his bedside, she told him, "I don't know if you remember what your doctor said, Aaron. He said he can't do anything curative now, only treat your pain."

"I remember," he replied. "That's okay. I've had a long enough life."

"Long," Yvonne said, "but was it good?"

He didn't answer, and Yvonne considered letting the conversation drop. Aaron had been taciturn even when his wife had been alive. But Yvonne realized that if she didn't get to know him better now, she never would.

She said, "Can I ask you another question?"

"Sure."

"Who have you been in your life?"

"That's a strange one. Nobody ever asked me that." He thought about it. "A housepainter. Damn good one."

"Anything more? I mean, you've been my uncle."

"Oh, yeah, an uncle, too. You've been a fine niece, Yvonne." A tear wet his cheek. He looked as though he was debating whether to say more. Yvonne waited.

Finally he said, "Did you know I was a father?"

"A father?"

"Two boys."

Yvonne was shocked. "I never knew you and Lynette had kids."

Aaron looked away. "They died. They were little when they died, of some genetic thing. It was before you were born. I guess your parents had their reasons for not telling you. I never mentioned it because I didn't want you to feel sorry for us. Our one little boy died, and the doctors encouraged Lynette and me to have another one. It was rare, they said; it'd never strike a family twice. But it did. The next little guy died, too."

Yvonne was too astonished to speak.

Aaron began to cry. Yvonne took his hand in hers. "He'd be sixty now, and his brother would be sixty-two. Old men. I think about them every day. That's the only father I could be to them, to just think about them all these years, have them live in me. I wonder if they'd be proud of me, their father, the painter." He wiped his eyes. "I guess I'll find out soon enough."

Aaron was able to find more meaning in his imminent transition by recognizing he'd been a father as fully, in his way, as he'd been a housepainter. Though my friend Ramona claims to have buried her archaic doormat version of herself, it's nonetheless permanently in her history, accessible should she ever need its healthier elements. Bonnie can still be high-powered when she needs to be and these days can voluntarily slow down and contemplate when that's called for. And even as Jim shifted into his next incarnation, he remained Jim the plumber, too: noticing a drip in his hospital room sink, he commented, "Needs an O-ring." We persist in what we were and we become more, too, which is why the process is called *growth*.

Although we culturally assume spiritual development to be a supernatural, ethereal process, it happens to be anything but. As a matter of fact, it's remarkably ordinary. According to Zen Buddhists, before enlightenment we chop wood and carry water, and after enlightenment, guess what? We chop wood and carry water. The world is still there as it was, but growth equips us better to relate to it. No matter how expansive our self-image, we must inevitably function in mundane life through mundane behavior. I might be a male and a carpenter and a Beethoven addict and meditator and sentient being and eternal soul and child of God, but I still have to stand in the kitchen and cook the kids' oatmeal.

TRANSFORMATION DAY BY DAY

It took at least our whole life for us to become who we are now, so we can't expect lightning-fast transformation. The most dramatic personal change is actually compounded of barely perceptible increments.

My friend Thad said, "You know, the first time my wife, Stephanie, went to a cancer support group, she didn't even stay. She told me she just sat there for ten minutes, all curled up, looking at the floor, and then she ran out. She came home and told me she couldn't go back.

"I asked her, 'Steph, what's that about? What'd it feel like being there, that you had to run out?' We talked about it for an hour, and I learned she was more frightened than I'd thought. She was scared of every unknown, scared of death, cancer, pain, tomorrow.

"I don't drop things easily. I let what she told me sit for a day and then I asked her, 'What is it about fear in general? Can you tell me more?'

"She said, 'All I know is that I hate fear. I don't want to be scared. I'm afraid of it.'

"I sat with that a minute and said, 'You know, Steph, some jazz musician said that Miles Davis was great because he was never afraid to be scared.'

"So I think it was Miles who got her back to that support group, maybe along with my agreement to go there with her. She told me on the way that she figured she was in nothing short of a life-and-death situation. She said, 'If I'm ever going to deal with my fears, here's my golden opportunity.'

"The first thing she told the other members was that she was scared. An older man, Lew, said, 'Stephanie, I appreciate your courage in saying that. We've all been scared. That's what cancer's about. But the more we talk about it, the less scared we are.'"

Stephanie told the group she had ovarian cancer that had seeded her lungs with tiny, inoperable tumors. She said she'd been given all the radiation she could take in her lifetime and was now finishing a round of chemotherapy her oncologist admitted was dubious.

Thad continued, "She cried as we left that meeting. I must've looked alarmed, because she told me, 'Don't worry, there's nothing wrong. I'm crying because I know I'm not alone. I always knew other people have cancer, too, but I didn't feel anyone truly understood me till tonight. God, that felt good.'

"During the next appointment with her oncologist, Steph complained of pain, but he acted like he hadn't heard her. She came home hurting more than ever and told me about it. I asked her, 'Honey, how'd you feel when that happened?'

"'In two words, plenty angry.'

"'What about it made you angry?'

"'Well, it felt like my pain didn't mean a thing to him.'

"'Uh-huh,' I said. 'I understand.'

"That annoyed her. She said, 'Oh, you understand? Well, let me ask you something, then, Thad. What would you have done?'

"I said, 'Well, since you ask, I guess I would've told him exactly what I thought was happening, that I didn't think he was taking me seriously. Then I would've told him how big the pain is, what it's doing to my life.'

"That took her by surprise, like maybe I actually did understand. I'd been going to her support group and listening, and I was actually learning something about coping with cancer. 'Oh,' she said. 'Yeah. That's definitely a good idea.' She made her anger work for her. She phoned the doctor right then, and he gave her a new prescription immediately.

"One night, when she told the support group she felt glum about her chances, Lew said, 'Yeah, at first I felt that way, too, but then I realized the disease has its odds but I'm in the equation, too. And since nobody can say for sure what'll happen to me, I may as well choose to believe what I like. My doc told me the chemo he wanted to try would have a 20 percent chance of working. So I said, "Well? What are you waiting for?" He looked at me funny and said, "Lew, I just told you there's only one chance in five the stuff will work. Why are you so eager?" I said,

"Hey, I just feel sorry for those other four dudes who ain't gonna make it.'"

"So Steph learned something about hope, really fierce hope. Maybe that allowed her to look at an even larger chunk of her fear. One day she told me, 'Thad, my cancer's a monster. It seems so huge and powerful that beside it I'm helpless. I need to find more strength than I have now.'

"I didn't know what to say to her. I wasn't sure where to find more strength for me, let alone for her. I couldn't help her, but she carried that wish around with her anyway, like a lock looking for a key.

"Funny, but she finally found the key in the most unlikely place, her oncologist's pessimism. That man never failed to give her a dose of gloom and doom. At one appointment he told her, 'Look, Stephanie, nobody beats this.' Another time he said, 'Stephanie, it won't help you to bury your head in the sand. This cancer will eventually take you out.'

"She spoke with me about that. She was reluctant to rebuke him directly because to a patient, a doctor's a powerful, intimidating figure. As she spoke to me about him, she found herself comparing him to her father, who wasn't the most encouraging person. Her father always told Steph what she couldn't do, never what she could. 'You can't dance,' he'd say. 'You can't draw.' 'You'll never be good at math.' And it was strange, because to hear her tell it, she showed him up every time, every time. Talking with me, Steph wondered if her father had done that deliberately, if maybe he knew his negativity would goad her into achieving.

"All that was quite an earful for me. I didn't know what to make of it. I only said, 'Hmmm.'

"As time went on, the doctor's despair actually began to amuse Steph. She'd come home from a visit and imitate him.

'Oh, Stephanie,' she'd say, 'this test looks terrible. As your doctor, I advise you not to buy green bananas.' Or, 'Bad news, Stephanie. You're more than 50 percent tumor, so you're no longer eligible to vote.'

"One visit, he said, 'Oh, I'm afraid the ship's beginning to sink, Stephanie. Your last pulmonary function test shows your breathing capacity's only 40 percent of normal.'

"She came home fuming. 'Forty percent!' she yelled. 'I'll show him.' She cashed in her inheritance from her grandfather and took me on a two-week tour of England and France. She made it a special point to climb to the top of Saint Paul's and Nôtre Dame. She had to prove him wrong. The week after we returned home, she insisted he repeat her pulmonary test. Now it showed 56 percent.

"She rubbed the doctor's nose in her tiniest victories. One morning, after she completed a three-mile hike in two hours, she phoned him. I heard her tell him, '. . . furthermore, I'm going to live as though I've been healed.'

"She told me he replied, 'Oh, I wouldn't want to hold out false hope, Stephanie.' But at that point I began to think he was on to her game. In fact, at her next appointment he told her, 'Frankly, Stephanie, I'm scared *not* to give you bad news.'

"But there finally came the day when he told her he'd done everything he could against the cancer, that further treatment would harm her more than help. That wasn't my favorite day. When she came home, we both cried. Later, she gave me her determined look.

"'Okay, then, Thad,' she said, 'I'm going to have to go to the big guns.'

"'What are the big guns?'

"'Lifestyle. High quality's a pretty strong medicine, you know.'

"So she went full-force back into her life. She didn't make a secret of her cancer, but you might say she wore it as an accessory rather than a garment. If anyone asked, she told them she had cancer but was healed. That must've confused some people. What she meant was that she might not have control over her cancer, but she knew she'd always be able to tweak her attitudes and make the minute-to-minute decisions of life.

"She wasn't Superwoman, though. She'd get an occasional disappointing test result or hear one of her doctor's morbid comments, and that would raise her fear again. But now, rather than hiding it, she'd play it out, just plain be fearful. To me or to the support group, she'd express it until she was finished expressing it, and then it was gone.

"During the time we attended her support group, many newcomers joined. They had no idea how fearful Steph had been at her first meeting. They knew her only as this outrageous person whose treatment consisted mainly of defying her disease and her doctor. When a new member asked Steph oh-so-delicately if she felt she might be in the teeniest bit of denial, she straightened up and proudly answered, 'Yes, of course I am. It's the only medicine that works for me now.'

"One evening, a young man came for the first time. He sat quietly in the circle and didn't look up. He looked like he was about to cry. I wondered if he'd bolt out, as Steph had done on her first visit. But he'd picked the seat beside her, so I might have seen it coming. Without a word, she reached down and took his hand, and he stayed.

"When Steph was first diagnosed, her doctor told her she probably wouldn't live past four months. I now believe that the old Steph died at four months and the new one was born then.

She led a full life, Steph did, and she died twenty-seven months after she was diagnosed. What a treasure she was. What a treasure she left me with."

As a model of transformation, what can Stephanie teach us? What does her example offer other sick people and their friends and relatives? After all, Stephanie wasn't cured. Nor can we prove she survived longer than others with similar diagnoses; she lived beyond the average for her type of cancer, but by statistical definition so do half of all patients. It seems evident that Stephanie did something dramatic and even arguably medicinal, but precisely what was it?

Compare who she was when we first met her with who she became. Initially crippled by fear, she gradually amassed impressive courage. Whereas at first she was helplessness itself, she became a model of creative control. Like a modern alchemist, she transformed her doctor's pessimism into a healing tonic, her despair into confidence. Stephanie used her illness to renovate her personhood.

This would have been a mortally difficult task had she been alone. On the spiritual path, support from others makes all the difference. Folksinger U. Utah Phillips tells an instructive story about support. He claims to know why circus accidents, once rare, are so common today. What's changed, he points out, is that circuses' live bands have largely been replaced by recordings. The high-wire artists of yesteryear moved according to their own timing, and the musicians below them adjusted their tempo accordingly. Today the artists' timing is secondary; following the music rather than leading it, they're more likely to move before they're ready. Artists perform more safely, in other words, when they're literally supported by an engaged orchestra. Stephanie's orchestra consisted of Thad and her support group, a community of people who understood her and whom she trusted enough to express herself ever more deeply.

OUTCOME

Can we guarantee every sick person benefits like Stephanie's? Of course not. Like the center of other existential issues, ultimate outcome is hidden in mystery, too. We can't know whether your sick friend or relative will live some given duration, gain equanimity or perhaps wisdom, transform himself, or, for that matter, reap any benefit whatever.

Mystery forces a standard deal on us: we must *accept* that we can never know outcomes in advance. That acceptance is more than an affirmation to stick on our refrigerator: it means giving up striving for some particular result. At the very least, to reach for a goal is to orient oneself toward the future, diverting attention from the present.

But there's even more at stake. I cautioned earlier in this book against attempting to fix the sick person. Of all the reasons to avoid fixing, the best is mystery's role: since we can't know what his outcome will be, we can't know what constitutes his "fix." "Have no appointments," Swami Satchidananda advised, "and you'll have no disappointments." Besides, truth be told, we hope too low as often as too high. When I've been able to resist expectations, sometimes results surpassed anything I would've hoped for.

TO HEAL

1. *Encourage your sick friend or relative to take his existential questions seriously.* Gently guide him if necessary.

(continued)

"Does your sickness make sense to you?" "Where do you find the strength to deal with it?"

2. Help him focus on the present rather than the past or future. Avoid "Why do you think you got sick?" and "How do you think things will go?" Ask instead, "Are you learning anything from all this?"

3. Don't push him into spirituality. If he's to genuinely transform, he'll do it not from your direction or his grim determination, but naturally, easily, as a result of his steadily growing self-image. Ask him occasionally, "How has your sickness changed you?"

4. Avoid attachment to outcome by keeping your own focus on the present. Accepting that the future's unknowable, recognize any preferences you have—about what he needs to do, what will happen to him, whether he'll transform himself—and then drop those preferences.

EIGHT

HEALING YOURSELF

> *The more you heal yourself, the more you can heal others; the more you heal others, the more you yourself are healed.*

There are so many things we are capable of, that we could be or do. The possibilities are so great that we never, any of us, are more than one-fourth fulfilled.

—Katherine Anne Porter

To live fully is to let go and die with each passing moment, and to be reborn in each new one.

—Jack Kornfield

GIVING WITHOUT END

My friend Curtis is a locally renowned healer who simply holds his hands on people for an hour. They shudder, cry, then relax and often fall asleep. When they awake, they feel dramatically better.

Curtis told me, "I saw Sarah for her emphysema last week. Before then my day was wild, so by the time I treated her and got ready to leave, I was pretty tired. On my way out, though, I noticed that Bernie looked under the weather, too, so I treated him. When I finally got home, I was a total wreck."

The next day Bernie, Sarah's husband, told me a slightly different story. "Curtis came to give Sarah a treatment," he said. "I wasn't sure how well he'd do, since he was obviously frazzled when he arrived. When he finished, I was relieved more for him than for Sarah. I hoped he'd go home and get some rest. But no, he had to treat me, too. He insisted, and I thought it'd be impolite to refuse him."

If you're going to heal sick people, you'll need to take better care of yourself than Curtis does. I don't mention this solely out of concern for your welfare, but for that of the sick people you attend as well: the quality of your encounter with them depends a great deal upon your condition.

Caregivers—both professionals and friends and relatives of sick people—commonly agree that they need to do for themselves what they do for others, yet they too often act otherwise. They give and give until they have nothing left, and then they give a little more. On any day, I can name for you a half-dozen healer friends who are all but burnt to ash and another score who are actively smoldering.

Curtis, who would be the first to admit he should take better care of himself, nevertheless focuses exclusively on others. My doctor friends tell me they'll slow down and nurture themselves as soon as they get an hour or two. When I ask almost any frayed caregiver how she's doing, she's likely to answer, "Oh, I'm okay. *He's* the important one now." In ignoring her own pain and fatigue, she acts exactly like Curtis. You may feel *you'll* never act this way, but I need to warn you that you'll encounter compelling pressure in that direction, since as a culture we see healing as a sacrificial act.

We believe healing necessarily injures its practitioners. Consider how we train doctors. Every ten years, like clockwork, the media expose a perennial scandal, hospitals' practice of requiring interns and resident physicians to work dangerously long hours. Alarmed by the consequent hazard to patients if not to the doctors themselves, citizens wring their hands, write letters to op-ed pages, call for congressional hearings. And then, like a cicada visit, the horror stories go underground until their next cycle. That the situation has hardly changed in my lifetime suggests there's wide implicit acceptance of physician overwork.

Nor is this overwork limited to time alone. We typically assign healers inappropriate responsibility as well. Many years ago I taught a community college course entitled "The Philosophy of Health," designed to examine our basic notions about health and sickness. During one session each semester I had students role-play both patient and doctor. They'd already played "patient" in their lives, so that was easy for them. Since playing "doctor" was a fresh challenge, I was always amazed how credibly they did it. Afterward, we discussed how they'd felt in each role. They consistently remarked on the burden they'd sensed as "doctors." "While I wore that white coat," went a typical statement, "I felt like the patient dumped her whole life into my lap, and it was up to me to cure her or solve her problem. I wouldn't have felt 'professional' telling her that made me uncomfortable, or that I already had enough problems of my own. I felt like I had to look smart and competent no matter what."

When you work with sick people, you'll be tempted to fall into this very role. Over the short term it can feel great; people do indeed respect omniscience and infallibility. But enact the role long enough, and you'll eventually stagger between altruistic exhaustion and frank martyrdom and in that condition will benefit no one.

It's not that healing *doesn't* deplete us. It easily can, since it's emotional and therefore energetic work. If we were perfectly tuned to the cosmos, ever-contoured to the flow of things, we'd need no restoration, but alas, we perform imperfectly from time to time, burn more calories than required. In the presence of sick people, we find our emotions yanking us about and our minds chattering more often than we'd like. We think too much, we gasp, get tight, hold our breath. Little wonder we're tired afterward, as though we'd transfused the sick person with our own blood and are now drained in the same measure she's healed. Feeling this way, we can reasonably conclude that our work as healers *will* necessarily wear us down.

Within that view, we're a kind of battery, a container of limited energy. Use it up, and there's nothing left. But some batteries are rechargeable, so imagine us as a battery under continual charge. Instead of a container, then, perhaps we're a conduit, a channel through which energy flows. We're not doomed to fatigue and burnout as long as we recharge as we discharge, fill as we empty, care for ourselves while we care for others.

Healing Ourselves

If you consider yourself a caregiver, I'll wager you didn't decide to become one overnight. Almost without exception, caregivers have a lifelong history of caring for others, sometimes to the point that they imagine self-care to be selfish.

Yet, ironically, the only way you can sustain your work is by taking care of yourself. In this quintessentially low-tech effort, you yourself are the total technology: you're not just reading *The Healing Companion*—you *are* the healing companion.

In his late eighties, Pablo Casals was asked why he, arguably the world's finest cellist, still practiced hours a day. He replied, "I think I'm beginning to make progress." Whatever progress you'll make begins now and remains a lifelong commitment. I'll discuss several areas in which you and I need to take care of ourselves, including

- increasing self-acceptance,

- achieving internal silence,

- developing comfort with uncertainty,

- accepting death,

- acknowledging our own suffering,

- recognizing our limits.

INCREASING SELF-ACCEPTANCE

My friend Flo is a single mother. When her ten-year-old son, Mark, suffers his occasional episodes of asthma, Flo sits with him until he's comfortable, sometimes a full twenty-four hours.

When he awoke late one night after coughing himself to sleep, he said, "Mom, what are you doing here? Why don't you get some rest?"

She answered, "I'd hate for you to wake up and not find me beside you."

"Mom, I'm okay. Please go to bed."

Flo answered, "What kind of a mother would I be if I slept while my son was sick?"

Like many of us, Flo is her own worst critic. Caregivers commonly suspect that unless they devote their lives to the sick person, they're callous or inept. Too often we leave a healing encounter mumbling to ourselves that we should have loved more and spoken less. Having fallen short of the ideal, we feel guilty rather than fulfilled. Physicians are hardly an exception to this rule. I don't think nonmedical people appreciate the extent to which doctors revisit every detail of their contacts with patients and lambaste themselves over suspected errors.

I believe inappropriate self-criticism is an endemic social disease. Beginning in childhood, we absorb subtle messages that our efforts don't quite suffice. We left our room dirty, should've offered our candy to our friends, could've diagrammed that sentence better. These little digs gradually summate in a background hum of assumed personal defect.

There are grounds for this conclusion since we do, after all, make mistakes. We're essentially imperfect. On the other hand, imperfection happens to be the highest state we human beings can achieve. We can relate to this paradox in a couple of ways. We can whip ourselves relentlessly for not being better than we can possibly be, or we can lighten up and be first in line for our own mercy.

An older friend put it well when, as he served his first rhubarb pie, he explained, "Well, here it is. I'd have made it better if I'd known how." That's true of our every act. I've behaved in ways I now consider stupid, even cruel, but now I know better. Knowing better means I manifest not only a bit more wisdom these days, but also a bit more compassion, forgiving myself for my past imperfections and for the current ones I don't yet recognize.

My seventy-six-year-old friend Penny said, "At my age, people get sick a lot. I haven't, but most of my friends are in and out of the hospital. I love to help them and do what I can. I'm not much good at sitting and listening, but people have always loved my cooking, so that's what I do.

"I recently realized, though, that something about it bothered me. I'd drop off a casserole and drive home feeling guilty. I'd think to myself, *There must be more I can do.* I know people who go along on doctor visits, sit at bedsides for hours, research medical information. I began to think that since I hadn't done any of that, I was falling short.

"A couple of days ago I took a pot of soup to Aggie, who had just come home after hip surgery. I put it in her fridge and poked my head into her room to say hello. She said, 'Penny, why do you look so terrible?'

"'Me, terrible?' I said. 'You're the one who just had surgery.'

"'Yeah,' she said, 'but you look kind of, well, guilty, like maybe you were making off with my silverware.'

"So I told Aggie how I felt. I sat down and said, 'Well, yes, I do feel guilty, but not because I took your silverware. It's because soup's not enough. I ought to be able to sit here with you or knit you a quilt or do something more than just cook. I feel like I don't do enough for my friends.'

"She got such a look on her face. 'I don't believe it,' she said. 'You do so much. Here, heat up that soup and let's eat it together and I'll tell you what a fine person you are. I know you won't want to hear that, but I'll tell you anyway. Maybe if you hear it enough, you'll stop beating yourself up.'

"So we ate my soup. What I learned from our conversation was that I accept criticism more easily than praise; it's hard for me to hear what a good friend I am. She said I just need practice—that maybe if I hear that from enough people I trust, I'll begin to believe it. Well, maybe she's right."

Since individuals are inevitably social, self-acceptance isn't simply narcissistic navel-gazing. Whether we mean to or not, we continually obey the Golden Rule, treating others exactly the way we feel about ourselves. While a positive self-image will generate loving relationships, a negative one will push toward criminality. Fortunately, society influences the individual, too: when others love us, our level of self-love rises. Like the sick people with whom we work, we blossom when we're valued or even honestly witnessed.

ACHIEVING INTERNAL SILENCE

The quiet mind we use to heal others gives us peace as well. Try this: close your eyes and pretend you're walking through a dense forest on a moonless night. You hear ominous snorts and growls nearby. You recall a recent newspaper story about wolf attacks. You stop. You try to peer into the darkness and then recall that wolves not only run faster than you but see better in the dark . . .

As you read that last paragraph, what happened to your breathing? Did your muscles tighten? Since the body responds physically to thoughts, we can run ourselves ragged even while sitting still. Sometimes edginess is helpful—say, when we're walking through a dark, wolf-infested forest. But more often than not, it occurs unconsciously when we have no use for it and so simply tires us. Our challenge, then, is to learn to operate our mind voluntarily instead of letting it operate us.

My friend Tim said, "I first got interested in being with sick people when my wife Rene was dying four years ago. A hospice nurse named Eileen came every couple of days and sat with Rene and just listened to her. Rene told Eileen more than she ever told me, and I got to feeling kind of jealous.

"One day when we were alone, I asked Rene why she spoke so

freely to Eileen and not to me. She said, 'Honey, I'd like to be that open with you, too, but you're always preoccupied. Whenever you're with me, there's some chore you need to do. Your eyes dart around. You can't wait to get on to the next project. When Eileen sits with me, she's not about to jump up and run out. She's so solidly present, I feel encouraged to say things I've never said before.'

"The next time Eileen came, I watched her. I hate to say it, but Rene was right. Eileen was as steady as a rock. She really did put all her attention into Rene. I couldn't do that any more than I could run a marathon. That wasn't who I was. As Eileen was leaving, I asked her how she did it, and she told me she'd actually learned it in classes. That sounded strange to me. Do we need to be trained to listen?

"Six months after Rene died, a friend from work got sick. When I visited him, I realized I was as preoccupied as I'd ever been with Rene. Right away, I didn't like that. Having seen Eileen work, I began to think maybe I could learn how to do what she did. I phoned the hospice and spoke with Eileen about it. She recommended I take their volunteer training.

"I jumped at it. Eileen had done so much for Rene, I wanted to learn how to be that good at listening. Well, they taught me how. I'm a hospice volunteer now, doing respite work. When I show up, the relatives can leave for a few hours and I sit at the bedside and listen. I'm not as good as Eileen, but I'm learning. I really am quieter, and people do notice it and speak to me more freely. I wouldn't have believed it."

One way you can move toward greater silence is to take training, as Tim did. Or you might want to review the exercise in chapter 3. Meditation, a formal self-quieting discipline, is becoming so popular in the United States that someone probably offers a course near you. Failing that, consult your library. I recommend two books in particular, Lawrence LeShan's *How to Meditate* (Little, Brown, 1999) and Jon Kabat-Zinn's *Full Catastrophe Living* (Delta, 1990). Bookstores generally carry a selection of effective meditation audiotapes as well, including my own *Transforming Your Chronic Pain* (New Harbinger, 1992).

DEVELOPING COMFORT WITH UNCERTAINTY

Your sick friend or relative can't know why she got sick, whether healing will come, or what her healed state might look like. Uncertainty is sickness' very atmosphere, and hers can whip her into such an emotional froth that she'll seek refuge in almost anything that looks like fact. That's why an undiagnosed disease is generally more distressing than one finally labeled, no matter what that label is. "At least," she'll say, "I know what I'm dealing with now."

Her uncertainties will likely make you uneasy, too. But while hers will ultimately resolve, you'll collect more as you spend time with sick people. Whatever discomforts those uncertainties hold for you will accumulate. That begins to be unhealthy, so you'll need to find a way to develop comfort with the vaguenesses that pervade sickness.

Consider your discomfort with uncertainty a phenomenon similar to your sick friend or relative's illness. Recall from chapter 2 that she doesn't suffer from her physical disease as much as from the meanings she's made of it—what I called her *illness*. In the same way, your current discomfort doesn't arise from anyone's physical situation but from your own thoughts about it, the meanings you've attached to it. The query "What's on your mind?" is particularly apt here: by definition, nothing can bother you except what's on your mind. That is, your discomfort is a product of, and exists in, your own mind. Please note well that I'm not saying, "It's all in your mind," as though your meanings are hollow fantasies. I've indicated repeatedly in this book that inasmuch as we're inescapably guided by our beliefs, they're very real indeed, and of paramount significance.

So once you notice you've been preoccupying yourself with speculations about the sick person's prognosis or her relationships or the side effects of her treatment, remind yourself that the preoccupation is yours. This isn't about her. It's about you.

Henry and Edna had been married fifty-five years when Henry learned he had prostate cancer. His doctor told him that tests indicated that his cancer was a slow-growing type. Not only did Henry have a far greater chance of dying of something else, the doctor said, but at his age the hazards of treatment posed a greater threat than the cancer.

Henry reflected, "I felt relieved, actually. I wasn't looking forward to surgery or radiation or hormones, so that took a load off my mind."

Edna, however, wasn't reassured in the least. "How can the doctor say that?" she asked Henry. "You have cancer, a life-threatening disease. How can he decide to do nothing?"

"I told you," Henry answered. "He pointed out that my age is even more life threatening. He said he'll monitor the cancer. If it looks like it's accelerating, he'll treat me."

"But I don't understand why he doesn't treat you now and wipe it out. How does he know the treatment will be more dangerous than the disease?"

Henry said, "Honey, I'm beginning to think our problem isn't so much my cancer as your anxiety about it. What do you think?"

They discussed it at length. They'd never before spoken their feelings about aging, getting sick, and losing each other.

Gradually, Edna came to terms with these eventualities. Now, two years later, she says, "I realize that when I insisted a while back that Henry get treated I was really saying how I couldn't accept losing him. Ever. I still feel that way, and at the same time I know it'll happen, one way or the other. I think something's happened to my priorities. Fearing for Henry isn't as gratifying as just loving him."

Your sick friend or relative may even borrow some of your increasing comfort with unknowns to relieve her unease.

My friend Audrey said, "My sister-in-law Kate's cancer has been in remission for five years now. Her doctor told her early on that a five-year remission is considered a cure. I've had cancer myself, so I don't think any number's magical. Five years' survival is terrific, but you can't ever be sure anybody's cured. That fact initially drove me nuts, but I felt better when I realized that nobody, anywhere, can know for sure they're cancer-free. People who've never been diagnosed with anything might have a few abnormal cells cooking away. We all have to live with that.

"Anyway, when I visited Kate she seemed terribly nervous. She was just about to have one of her 'routine' periodic exams. She knows pretty much what to expect in the exam; it's waiting for the results that gives her the willies. When you've had cancer, you may as well throw out the word *routine* since almost anything can look like a crisis.

"She kept asking me, 'What if he finds a recurrence?' and 'What if such-and-such a blood test is abnormal?' and 'What if he finds a totally new cancer?' She took each of those questions and ran all the way with it. 'If I have a recurrence, then I'll get chemo, which'll make my hair fall out and I've already given away my wig, so I won't be able to go to my reunion.' 'Who'll bring me food? I hate it when other people shop for me. They buy all the wrong stuff.' And so on, and so on. She was making us both crazy.

"Making oneself crazy is something I'm already good at, thank you. When I was getting treated, I mentally suffered every possibility and then some, splattered my mind all over the walls, and you know what? The reality was never as horrible as my imagination predicted. I finally saw a counselor to learn how to settle myself down.

"I told Kate all that, but it didn't make any difference. And I certainly couldn't assure her that her fantasies *weren't* going to happen, since no one knows. All I could do was sit there while she awfulized. After a while, she noticed I hadn't said anything. She said, 'Audrey, don't you care?'

"I said, 'Hey, of course I care. I love you. But you're not talking about what's going on now. You're chattering about the future, and pretty pessimistically, I might add. You're suffering from anxiety, not cancer. It's your mind that's whipping you around. And that's normal. It happens with cancer. I know. I've done my share.'

"She heard that. She said, 'Well, I guess you're right. But how can I stop doing it?'

"I had her sit down, close her eyes, and watch her breath. I breathed along with her. 'Look,' I said, 'this is how you're breathing.' She was panting like a puppy, and she didn't realize it till she stopped and paid attention. 'Try slowing down,' I told her. 'I'll slow down, and you breathe along with me.'

"It wasn't easy for either of us. One look at her, and I got nervous, too, so I had to keep centering myself, maintain a slow, calm breath. It took fifteen minutes, but when she was finally able to do it, she brightened up. She said, 'Wow, Audrey! I'm not nervous now.'

"She thought it was magic. She had me come back the next couple of days and do it again with her till she could learn to do it for herself. At this point she thinks maybe she has a decent handle on her anxiety."

I've discussed uncertainty as though the distress it creates is a foregone conclusion. Actually, a fair number of people accept it rather easily, and a few others are positively exhilarated by it. The late comedienne Gilda Radner said, "Life is about not knowing, having to change, taking the moment and making the best of it, without knowing what's going to happen next. Delicious ambiguity."

ACCEPTING DEATH

The more sick people we contact, the more impossible it becomes to evade the issue of death. In our daily lives, where death isn't conspicuous, we can afford to ignore it. But when we sit regularly at bedsides, it's sure to tug at our elbow. We may find ourselves listening to our sick friend or relative when suddenly our mind mutters, "How much more can she waste away? What if she dies? She can't die on me. Death is scary/awful/disgusting. If she dies, has my work been for nothing? At least *I'm* not dying now. Will I die this way?" Of course, while we're attending this gripping monologue of ours, we can't hear *her*.

Even if we regather our wits during this particular encounter, that sort of chatter is sure to arise again unless we eventually deal with the issue. And the issue isn't her death or, for that matter, death at all, but our thoughts tangent to our own death.

"Dying doesn't bother me," a man with advanced cancer told me. "I'm just afraid of all the rang-dang-doo I'll have to go through to get there." He echoed what I'd heard from numerous others. When we get right down to it, death doesn't frighten us nearly as much as the weighty uncertainties that precede and follow it. That is, death can seem bigger than life, so to speak, because it's the mother of all uncertainties.

Helping you thoroughly confront your eventual death is beyond the scope of this book, but certainly you can begin to do so by learning to meditate. Controlling your mental chatter, you'll face the issue in relative equanimity, and only then will benefits accrue. I've learned that calm attention to my mortality continually improves my life. Hundreds of people with life-threatening disease have taught me that when we take our impermanence seriously, we begin to act more from conscious choice than from numb habit. In her seminal work *On Death and Dying*, Dr. Elisabeth Kübler-Ross concluded that once we've addressed the emotions around our own death, we stop clinging to life and live it instead. As healers, that means we can withdraw our attention from death as the obligatory enemy and place it instead in our sick but unquestionably living friend or relative.

Marguerite said, "I sat with my grandmother while she was dying.

"She said, 'I'll miss you, Marguerite. I've always loved you, you know.'

"I said, 'Oh, Grandma, you're not going anywhere.'

"She looked at me like I was crazy. 'Marguerite,' she said, 'don't you know I'm dying?'

"That sounded so morbid. I said, 'Nothing of the sort, Grandma. You'll live past a hundred.'

"But my grandmother was always kind of stern with me. She said, 'Marguerite, repeat after me: Grandma, you're dying, and it's okay.'

"Gulp. I couldn't do it. So she said it again. I made myself repeat it. 'Grandma, you're dying, and it's okay.'

"She said, 'See? Nothing's changed. No bolt of lightning. I'm still here and we still love each other, but now you know we won't be here together forever.'

"I said to myself, *It's true. She really is dying. I don't like it, but something about that really is okay, like it makes her life complete.* From then until she died, we both managed to be absolutely honest. Of all the things Grandma did for me, that was one of the best."

ACKNOWLEDGING OUR OWN SUFFERING

We can heal others to the extent we've felt and expressed our own suffering. Conversely, people who pretend invulnerability don't make good healers.

My friend Milt told me, "Not long ago I ran into a guy named Charlie in a bar. He and I had worked together twenty-five years back. First thing he said was 'Milt, I have lung cancer.'

"What do you say to something like that? Actually, I resented him for telling me. I mean, after not seeing somebody all those years, the first thing you say is a bummer like that? So I said, 'Hey, hang in there, man,' and I made my way out. I haven't seen him since.

"Last year, Elise, next door, came down with some kind of kidney disease. She got so depressed, she had to go on pills, and so did her husband, Ben. I've never seen such a down household. It made me and Cindy so uncomfortable we didn't even want to borrow sugar from them.

"Well, it's funny how the world works. Two months ago, Cindy got breast cancer. She was really torn up emotionally. But what shocked me almost as much as her diagnosis was that I was devastated, too, maybe even more. I'd never imagined anything could affect me like that. Cindy wound up handling it okay, but I eventually had to go on antidepressants. It was needing those pills that finally opened my eyes. I hadn't really known before how Charlie or Elise or Ben felt, and now I couldn't avoid it. Turns out it's a pretty deep business.

"Cindy had surgery and chemo, and it looks like her treatment's working. But her cancer never bothered us a tenth of what the emotional roller coaster did. We'd cry, then get angry, then get depressed. It was a terrible ride. Now when my friends tell me they're sick, I hear them differently. You can't truly be there for anybody unless, well, you've been there yourself."

However we've been wounded—sick, injured, abused, or even hurting as a result of pain around us—we're still not immune to the subtle cultural mandate to keep it to ourselves and look strong.

My friend Zena said, "It was really hard on me, having George sick. I couldn't be myself. I felt wrecked, but I didn't want to cry in front of him. I thought it'd only make him feel worse.

"Our daughter Libby visited from California. The way she tells it, people cry openly there at bus stops and in supermarkets. I asked her how crying would help. She said, 'Mom, your body can't lie. Dad can see how you feel and how you're holding it in, too, so you're not gaining anything. Not crying is only separating the two of you.'

"She had a point. Holding it in made me miserable and I couldn't do it much longer, anyway. So I finally cried in front of George. Just as I had feared, that made him cry. Well, the cat was out of the bag then, so we cried together. And Libby was right. When we finally finished crying, it was like clouds lifting after a rainstorm. We felt so much closer and easier with each other. Now I show George whatever I'm feeling, and it turns out he's usually feeling that way, too."

One way to sense your own woundedness in a healing encounter is to hear the sick person's story emotionally. As I suggested more fully in chapter 5, sense her with your heart as well as your ears and eyes. Steve Sanfield, a professional storyteller, granted me his secret for getting his audience to do that. "When I was a novice," he said, "I began stories with 'Once upon a time.' That works, but it doesn't engage listeners as deeply as 'Do you remember . . . ?'"

By opening with that phrase, he invites his audience to pluck feelings from their physical cache. When they do that, his story feels to them less like it's coming from him than from their own insides. We can listen in a similar way by matching our own suffering to the sick person's. Do you remember . . .

My friend Marty said, "My father had what was called a minor stroke. The first time I visited him in the hospital, I held his hand and thought, *Oh, poor Dad.* He's a retired English teacher, so I knew his inability to speak couldn't have been minor to him.

"Seeing the fear in his eyes reminded me of my own experience when I was four years old. I'd been running with a lollipop in my mouth. I tripped and fell on my face, and the stick injured the back of my throat. My father sped me to the hospital. What a mess! It bled a lot and swelled up so much that it was all I could do to breathe air in and out. I couldn't speak for maybe a week and was too young to write. I can't remember much else from when I was four, but my loneliness during that week remains crystal clear. I haven't taken speech for granted since. We have these things we want to say, need to say, and when we can't get them out it's like we're buried alive.

"When I remembered that at Dad's bedside, suddenly the picture looked different to me. He was locked away alone, and believe me, I knew how he felt. My heart just shot out to him. I cried and hugged him. He knew I understood what he was going through, and it seemed that gave him relief. Actually, he told me exactly that a month later, when he began to get his speech back."

RECOGNIZING OUR LIMITS

Frankly, not even saints are always in a healing mood. Your sick friend might want you to attend her, but you just heard your spouse has been fired, so you'd rather go home. Or maybe you're put off by the crowd carousing around her bed. Or you're just plain tired.

So before you go to heal anyone, assess yourself. Do you feel up to it? If you don't, say so. Simply not feeling in a healing mood is adequate reason not to visit a bedside. You don't have to give a reason, or for that matter even know the reason. The feeling is good enough: if the sick person's a genuine friend, she'll love you no matter what you do.

In addition to your personal limits, there's the ultimate limit inherent in healing itself: *you can't know what you've accomplished.* Human influence is trivial compared with that of the inscrutable cosmos, so for all your efforts, healing still comes from grace. When your sick loved one feels better, is it a result of your encounter, or would that have happened anyway? If her suffering remains unrelieved, did you fail, or would she have felt even worse if not for your intervention? You don't know, and you can't know. Your job is only to stir the pot; you're never wholly responsible for the flavor.

This ineluctable blind spot can vex you, leave you always wondering whether you could've done more. Repetitive self-doubt is an erosive practice, so in each situation you'll have to find a balance between effort and humility, your active intervention along with detachment regarding outcome.

The boundary between what we can accomplish and what grace provides is where we can touch the Divine. Whole religions are built on the union of action with deliberate nonaction. Christian theology advises that we must die to be reborn, that we get by giving up. Zen Buddhists discover the meaning of their koan, their insoluble riddle, only when they abandon their logical search for it. The word *Islam* literally means "surrender."

Healing requires exactly this union. We actively create a healing atmosphere by sitting with the sick person, asking her questions, and listening carefully. Then, aware that the universe creates its own justice, we can do no more other than to let go, accede to what's to be.

One afternoon my friend Marcella became inexplicably dizzy and disoriented. Her husband, Orv, rushed her to their doctor, who, alarmed, hospitalized her immediately. Marcella gradually lost consciousness. A consulting neurologist determined that she had acute encephalitis, a brain infection caused by a virus. He initiated aggressive treatment, but Marcella continued to decline. Twenty-four hours later, she was comatose and her pupils were fixed and dilated, a grave sign. Orv summoned their priest to give her last rites.

Father Luke arrived at Marcella's bedside. "Orv," he said, "would you like to pray with me?"

"Let's pray she lives, Father."

"You do that, Orv. That's good. But there's only one thing I ever pray for—that God's will be done."

They prayed together then, and Father Luke gave Marcella last rites as Orv had requested.

Then she unexpectedly stabilized. The staff maintained her life support and fed her intravenously the next two weeks. One morning while Orv was present, Marcella blinked her eyes. By later in the day it was evident she was responding to questions with eye-blinks.

Excited by Marcella's progress, Orv phoned Father Luke. "I

think my prayers have been answered, Father," Orv said. "It looks like she's pulling out of this, like she'll live."

Two days later, Marcella was sitting up and conversing, and in a week she was able to go home in a wheelchair. Over the following months, she patiently learned to walk again. But she increasingly noticed a troubling void. "It felt like encephalitis erased so much of my history," she said much later. "Whoever I'd been before was gone, and I wasn't sure who I was now."

Speaking extensively with Orv about this vague feeling, she came to sense a strange excitement in it. "If I'm not sure who I am now, I guess I'm free to be whoever I want," she said. Over months, she developed interests and friendships she'd never had before her sickness. She took up the violin, joined a book group, worked on a friend's city council campaign.

Now, a year later, Orv says, "Marcella's an entirely different person than she was before her encephalitis. She didn't just survive it. She's more vibrant than ever, what I'd call a born-again human being.

"When Father Luke dropped by a few days ago, he asked me, 'Orv, do you remember what we prayed for at Marcella's bedside?'

"I thought back to it. 'I wanted her to live,' I said, 'and I'm grateful my prayer was granted. But you prayed for something different, didn't you?'

"He reminded me that he'd prayed God's will be done. I've been thinking about that since then. To put it mildly, I suspect there's more going on than I know about."

To be passionate in our healing work and dispassionate toward its results doesn't mean resigning ourselves to any lesser outcome. On the contrary, we're opening ourselves to every outcome. All we're giving up is our preconceptions, admittedly a difficult task, but one that sometimes allows a grander healing than we might've imagined.

HEALING AS ORDINARY

Healing is a spiritual process, literally marvelous. And at the same time it's nothing special.

Of course, it seems special at first, possibly because in these times common intimacy truly is uncommon. But as we continue to engage in it mindfully, it gradually becomes our natural style rather than the application of an extraneous skill. We finally find ourselves being compassionate even when we hadn't intended, and at that point healing is no longer anything special to us.

I don't depict healing as ordinary to degrade our efforts, but actually to praise us for having raised our standards. When healing's intimacy looks *normal* to us, we'll see any lesser connection—say, habitually rushing around and barely contacting others—as undesirable if not intolerable. We'll naturally drift away from critics and pessimists and toward those who love us unconditionally.

With that shift, our own transformative journey commences. Its preparation began once we saw sickness as a reminder to reflect on our lives, mortality as a call to awaken to the moment, and suffering as an invitation to compassion.

TO HEAL

1. *Ask yourself if you're ready, willing, and able* before you agree to a healing encounter. If you're not, *for any reason*, say so and postpone it.

2. *Take care of yourself.* Since you yourself are healing's technology, your work will be as effective as your

physical and emotional condition. Your healing practice requires your *continual* self-care.

3. Increase your self-acceptance. You're a fallible human being, doing as well as you can reasonably do. When others love you and praise you, assume that their expressions are sincere.

4. Learn how to be quieter. Through meditation or some other appropriate discipline, develop progressively greater mental silence so you can devote fuller attention to sick people.

5. Increase your comfort with uncertainty. All you can do in response to the uncertainties that pervade sickness and healing is accommodate to them.

6. Feel, acknowledge, and address your own suffering. Listen to the sick person's illness story with your heart; that is, feel her suffering as though it's yours. It's all right to tell her your feelings. "Hearing you describe what you've been through, I feel sad."

7. Do your best and then let go. Be open to any possibility. You can't know the results of your work, and the ultimate outcome is out of your hands, anyway.

NOTES

FOREWORD

1. R. L. Golden, "William Osler at 150, an Overview of a Life," *Journal of the American Medical Association* 282(23) (December 15, 1999): 2252–58.

2. J. A. Astin, "Why Patients Use Alternative Medicine—Results of a National Survey," *Journal of the American Medical Association* 279(19) (1998): 1548–53.

CHAPTER ONE

1. C. Pert, M. Ruff, et al., "Neuropeptides and Their Receptors, a Psychosomatic Network," *Journal of Immunology* 135, suppl. 2 (August 1985): 820s–26s.

2. B. Horrigan and Candace Pert, "Neuropeptides, AIDS, and the Science of Mind-Body Healing," *Alternative Therapies* 1 (1995): 70–76.

3. C. Henderson, personal communication, September 20, 1999.

CHAPTER THREE

1. D. L. Rosenhan, "On Being Sane in Insane Places," *Science* 179 (January 1973): 250–58.

CHAPTER FOUR

I. William Masters and Virginia Johnson, *Human Sexual Response* (Little, Brown & Co., 1966), p. 311.

CHAPTER SIX

I. Richard Feynman, *The Pleasure of Finding Things Out* (Helix/Perseus Books, 1999), p. 146.